Paediatric Primary Health Care

4TH EDITION

Paediatric Primary Health Care

4TH EDITION

J.D. Ireland, D.J. Power, D.L. Woods & F. Desai

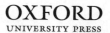

OXFORD
UNIVERSITY PRESS

0122I487

OXFORD
UNIVERSITY PRESS

Great Clarendon Street, Oxford OX2 6DP

Oxford University Press is a department of the University of Oxford.
It furthers the University's objective of excellence in research, scholarship,
and education by publishing worldwide in

Oxford New York

Auckland Cape Town Dar es Salaam Hong Kong Karachi
Kuala Lumpur Madrid Melbourne Mexico City Nairobi
New Delhi Shanghai Taipei Toronto

with offices in
Argentina Austria Brazil Chile Czech Republic France Greece
Guatemala Hungary Italy Japan Poland Portugal Singapore
South Korea Switzerland Thailand Turkey Ukraine Vietnam

Oxford is a registered trade mark of Oxford University Press
in the UK and in certain other countries

Published in South Africa
by Oxford University Press Southern Africa, Cape Town

Paediatric Primary Health Care 4th edition
ISBN 0 19 578404 9 (10-digit, current)
ISBN 978 0 19 578404 6 (13-digit, from 2007)
© DL Woods, JD Ireland, DJ Power, F Desai 2006

The moral rights of the author have been asserted
Database right Oxford University Press (maker)

First edition (*Notes on Primary Care for Paediatric Clinical Nurses* by JD Ireland,
DJ Power & DL Woods) published 1981 by the Department of Paediatrics and Child
Health, University of Cape Town. Second edition (*Paediatric Primary Care* by
JD Ireland, DJ Power & DL Woods) published in 1985 by College Tutorial Press. Third
edition (*Paediatric Primary Health Care* by JD Ireland, DJ Power, DL Woods &
DH Hoogenhout) published in 1994 by Oxford University Press Southern Africa.
Fourth impression published in 2001.

Fourth edition published 2006

Commissioning editor: Zarina Adhikari
Editor: Aimeé van Rooyen
Medical proofreader: Mary Hann
Designer: Brigitte Rouillard
Cover design: Brigitte Rouillard
Illustrator: Mary Hann
Indexer: Ethné Clarke

Published by Oxford University Press Southern Africa
PO Box 12119, N1 City, 7463, Cape Town, South Africa

Set by RHT desktop publishing, Durbanville
Printed by ABC Press, Cape Town

1 8 OCT 2006

Contents

Authors

J.D. Ireland MD (UCT), FCP (SA)
Associate Professor, Senior Lecturer and Senior Paediatrician
School of Child and Adolescent Health, University of Cape Town and Red
Cross War Memorial Children's Hospital

*D.J. Power MD (UCT), MBBS (London), MRCP (UK), DCH, RCP & S (UK),
DCM (UCT)*
Emeritus Professor
School of Child and Adolescent Health, University of Cape Town

D.L. Woods MD (UCT), FRCP (London), DCH, RCP & S (UK)
Emeritus Associate Professor and Honorary Neonatologist
Neonatal Medicine, School of Child and Adolescent Health, University of
Cape Town and Groote Schuur Hospital

*F. Desai RN, RM, BA (Comm Health, Nursing Education: UNISA), DNA
(UNISA), Paediatrics and Advanced Paediatrics and Neonatal Nursing
Science*
Deputy Director: Maternal, child, and women's health
Department of Health, Provincial Government of the Western Cape

Preface

More than ten years have passed since the publication of this manual – a period which has been witness to much change for children in South Africa. The country's commitment to this important group in society has been effected through ratification of the Convention on the Rights of the Child; inclusion of a special Bill of Rights for children in the South African Constitution; child-oriented legislative reform; and a series of policies and programmes which target the rights and needs of children. Among these, their rights to survival, development, and protection have been cornerstones which, along with children's rights to participation in decisions about their own lives, have informed strategies towards improving their lives and helping them to secure their rightful place in society.

The turn of the century was also marked by disillusionment that the global hope of health for all by the year 2000 had not been realised. Across the globe, there was agreement that revitalisation of the lofty goals of the Alma Ata Declaration on primary health care would have to take form in a series of focussed, substantive interventions to advance the health of all the world's children. This manual on *Paediatric Primary Health Care* has been an important contributor to these interventions.

Setting out in 1994 to make a real difference to children's health, the manual has achieved its goal on several fronts. Firstly, in focusing on those health conditions which account for the burden of death and disease of the majority of South Africa's child population, it has made a significant impact on national health priorities. Secondly, it aims to strengthen health care for children at the primary level, thus contributing to national efforts to promote access to health for everyone. Thirdly, in providing guidelines for essential health care through a system of management and referral, it gives effect to the country's commitment to providing effective care. And finally, it is an important manual for building on the knowledge and practice of those who care for children.

The manual is the result of experience of many teachers, learners, and practitioners from across the country, and improving on the first edition, this one is based on useful commentary from those who have used it as a teaching and learning resource in the last decade.

At a local level, I have been privileged to benefit from this manual as a child health teacher and practitioner. At a national level, I have also been concerned with matters of policy for children, plans for child health, and national strategies for human resource development. Against this background, I have no doubt that *Paediatric Primary Health Care* will continue to make a crucial contribution to the promotion of the health of South Africa's children, and the overall development of our country.

Marion Jacobs
Director: School of Child and Adolescent Health
University of Cape Town
2006

Introduction

Paediatric Primary Health Care serves several purposes. Firstly, it acts as a reference for doctors or nursing tutors who are currently training, or who wish to train Primary Care Paediatric Clinical Nurses. Secondly, it aims to help registered nurses (RNs) who, by force of circumstance, are already providing health care to children in unofficially extended roles and often without additional appropriate training.

This book will also be of use to those doctors and nurses responsible for providing a better health service to the children of southern Africa. It covers both common paediatric conditions and practical aspects of their management. These topics are often not easily found in the larger textbooks, and so this book serves as a handy reference for common paediatric problems. This makes it especially useful for medical students and for general practitioners interested and involved in the health care of children.

Primary health care for children: A new model

The problems involved in providing comprehensive medical care for all the citizens of a developing country are difficult and complex. In southern Africa, the quality of medical care ranges from very good to totally inadequate. The philosophy of the present services has up till now been that of a developed country. As such, its aim has been high quality care for the individual patient. It assumed that all patients are seen and largely managed by a doctor. This is simply not possible in developing countries, and alternative sources of health care are currently planned and used for southern Africa.

Those most at risk from inadequate health care provision are children. Their numbers, rural distribution, and vulnerability to inadequate nutrition and infection make them particularly susceptible to disease. The long-term consequences of insults to health in children affect their potential as adults, and this further emphasises the need to prioritise health care services for children. Because of the shortage and mal-distribution of doctors in southern Africa, such services require additional members of the health team with expanded roles.

Training RNs for this task has been shown to be a highly effective solution. By extending the role of nurses, they can provide many of the services traditionally considered the province of the doctor. RNs trained as Primary Care Paediatric Clinical Nurses can enable doctors in the areas of greatest need to play a different role. These doctors can thus be freed to act as teachers, organisers, supervisors, planners, and consultants to the health team. This will ensure that the special skills of the doctor are not swamped by an overwhelming patient load consisting of routine problems. The majority of these problems can be adequately dealt with by RNs, with the doctor acting as a consultant for selected specific problems. This allows for the appropriate use of the training and skills of health personnel in both categories.

The spectrum of disease in southern Africa is such that many of the conditions causing the greatest morbidity and mortality can effectively be treated if seen and diagnosed early. The nurse with additional training can competently manage most of the common problems of childhood on her or his own.

It is envisaged that the future health care service will use RNs in extended roles to a far greater extent than at present. They are the logical solution to the problem of the limited numbers of doctors and their serious maldistribution.

The nurse trained in this way will function as a nurse with an extended role. This concept is generally accepted. Once it is widely applied, the health care services will be immeasurably improved, and an appropriate health care service for the country will become a reality. If health personnel are used at the correct levels of skill and training, they will be better motivated and take pride in their achievements. Only by making full use of both the medical and nursing professions can adequate health care be provided for all the peoples of southern Africa. This will then be at a cost that the countries can afford. For this to succeed, it is vital that doctors recognise and support these principles, and participate both in training and their implementation.

Basic provision of services for children

Primary health care services for children are ideally provided at the same time and place as those for adults. Services should be comprehensive, which means offering preventive, promotive, and curative services at the same time and venue. The services may be based in a mobile clinic mainly run by nurses, or in a larger 'community health centre', which typically has at least some full-time doctors, therapists, simple laboratory and X-ray facilities, and 24-hour maternity and casualty services. These services may be publicly run, or be a function of a private body such as a health maintenance organisation. The services at a typical clinic or community health centre should include:

- Maternal health care.
- Child health care.
- HIV counselling, diagnosis, and treatment.
- Immunisation.
- Family planning.
- Tuberculosis testing and treatment.
- Sexually transmitted diseases: Testing and treatment.
- General outpatients.
- Geriatric and mental health services (in some areas).
- Information services, for example public health statistics.

Child health clinic procedure

In a comprehensively run service, there are no separate sessions to cater for 'well babies', immunisations, or infants. A patient's needs are met as and when they present. Often a crisis or acute illness prompts a parent to bring her child to the clinic. Health services need to be able to seize these opportunities for preventative care.

At each visit, a child and his or her parent or guardian should go through the following stages:

1. Registration and issuing of a Road to Health (RTH) card, if the child does not yet have one.
2. Weighing and charting of weight for age on the RTH card. This must be done every time the child visits the clinic, as it is an essential measure of the child's well-being.
3. Sick children must have their temperatures taken, and reception staff must enquire about vomiting. If the temperature is higher than 38 °C, collection of urine should begin while the child waits to be seen. If there is diarrhoea or vomiting, oral rehydration solution (ORS) should be given to the child at once.
4. Consultation with clinic sister or doctor. This may be for a specific complaint which involves an examination, or for routine advice and counselling. At all visits, the immunisation status and basic developmental progress should be assessed. Medication should ideally be issued directly by the consulting sister, who can discuss treatment with the patient, or patient's parents. Medication should be taken from a short, well-chosen list of medications, which should be used according to standard protocols agreed to by the local district health authorities.

5. Immunisations and treatments are carried out as indicated.
6. Issue or sale of subsidised milk and / or foods. This depends on what is locally available, but strict criteria must be laid down as to who should receive such foods, and under what circumstances.
7. Education: The visit should always involve education of the parents or guardian, in the form of talks, group discussions or demonstrations.

Nutrition clinics

Many clinics find it useful to have a weekly session for malnourished children. The activities of this service should include:

- Regular weighing and charting to assess progress.
- Screening for anaemia and TB.
- Investigation of social problems with referral to appropriate welfare agencies when necessary; for example:
  - Non-support.
  - Maintenance grants.
- Nutritional education in the form of individual advice, talks, group discussions, and demonstrations on the preparation and use of basic foodstuffs.
- The cheap (or possibly free) supply of basic foodstuffs, for example maize meal, beans, skim milk, and leafy green vegetables.

Records

The simplest and least expensive system of record-keeping is based on the Road to Health (RTH) card, which is kept at home by the parents and produced at each visit. This approach has been shown to be highly effective, and very few cards are lost by regular attendees. This system often has the back-up of a clinic-based card reminder system for the detection of immunisation and TB treatment defaulters.

Systems which involve keeping records at the clinic are more expensive in terms of both staff time and money, and are not necessarily more reliable or efficient.

Staffing

The role of doctors will depend on their availability. Where there are relatively few doctors in proportion to nurses or other clinical assistants, the doctor's function is to work alongside the nurses, see referrals, and act in a teaching / supporting capacity. If the ratio of doctors is more plentiful, they may undertake more consultations.

When trained nursing staff are in short supply, it is essential that tasks are delegated where appropriate to less trained staff. For example, trained auxiliaries can satisfactorily carry out the following clinic duties:

- Registration.
- Weighing and charting.

If possible, some staff must be allocated to home visiting. This may be to find newborn infants whose mothers have given birth at home, to trace defaulters and contacts, or to assess social circumstances. Trained community health nurses are ideal, but there are few of them and they can be expensive to employ. Community health workers can perform these duties.

Medication

The medications available for children at clinics should be limited to a short list agreed upon at district health authority level, and used according to mutually agreed protocols. In South Africa, these medications are on the Essential Drug List (EDL). Patients in need of more sophisticated therapy should be referred to the next level of care. Hospitals can supply clinics with other medicines for specific patients for dispensing on a long-term basis, for example in the case of cardiac or epileptic patients.

Emergencies

Ideally, space should be set aside in a clinic for emergencies. The necessary equipment and medications should be kept here, and must be quickly available. Staff must be trained and equipped to deal with:

- Dehydration / shock.
- Convulsions.
- Hypoglycaemia in the newborn.
- Resuscitation of the newborn.

Communication and transport

An essential part of primary health care is timeous upward referral. A communication system linked to the local transport centre or ambulance station is needed, together with an adequate supply of functioning ambulances, or other forms of transport. The lack of adequate communication and transport remains one of the biggest problems bedevilling primary health care services in developing countries.

ORT Corner

Every clinic should have an oral rehydration therapy (ORT) corner where dehydrated children can be observed.

History and physical examination

History-taking: General

To define and understand a patient's problem(s) requires three aspects of assessment: (a) history-taking; (b) physical examination; and (c) relevant investigations. Of the three, the history is the most important, especially so in paediatrics. Not only does it provide essential information regarding the present and related problems, it can also reveal other aspects of family and social circumstance, birth and development, immunisation status, previous illness, and other relevant problems. These may not be the reason for the present visit, but are essential for the comprehensive care of the patient.

It is essential to find out which language the person accompanying the child understands. If necessary, use a translator. This is very important as an incorrect history can be obtained if both parties do not fully understand each other.

Establishing a relationship

The first meeting between yourself and the parent or guardian, as well as the child (if old enough), establishes the basis of your future working relationship.

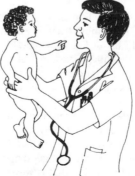

Figure 1.1 Establishing a relationship

Your conduct and manner determine whether such a relationship will be a friendly and productive one, or whether it will be neutral, guarded, or even negative and antagonistic. A friendly, interested, caring approach helps in many different ways. (A warm room that is child-friendly also assists in putting the parents and child at ease.) There is a tendency amongst doctors and nurses who are very busy and trying to cope with large patient loads, to use shortcuts by missing out details of history-taking. This is an incorrect and dangerous practice. Usually, more relevant information is obtained through the taking of a good history than by physical examination and laboratory or special investigations.

Listening to mothers

Because mothers are considered 'lay persons' and are seen to have limited medical knowledge, there is a tendency, especially by inexperienced staff, to assume that their assessment and interpretation are unimportant. Nothing could be more dangerous or unwise. A mother's insight, instinct, and intuition can only assist the medical assessment. Mothers are rarely wrong, but may express or interpret the problem according to their own experience, understanding, and emotional make-up. It is best to take careful note of what they say. However, the history may often be supplied by fathers, grandparents, guardians, friends, neighbours, older siblings, or through a translator. The reliability of such information may then vary greatly. The source and accuracy of such information must thus be taken into account.

Personalised approach

At the outset, introduce yourself by name and take the time (depending on the age of the child) to establish friendly verbal contact with the child, who is an individual in his or her own right. A few friendly questions or remarks will help the child relax and feel comfortable. Time spent 'making friends' will save time and effort when it comes to performing the examination, and allow for a more informative examination. Be sensitive to cultural differences.

The history should ideally be taken in private, but if there are other doctors, students, or nurses present, they should be introduced, and an explanation given as to why they are there. Let the mother talk while you direct the course of the conversation. A good opening is to ask her to tell you about her child and what it is that is worrying her. If after history-taking, examination, investigation, diagnosis, and management you have not specifically addressed what she was originally worried about, you will still have an unhappy and dissatisfied mother on your hands, even if your diagnosis and treatment are theoretically correct. Children have names and should be addressed or referred to accordingly. The name to which a child answers may be a pet name or a shortened version of the official birth name found in the folder. Address the child by this pet name, or a rather puzzled 'Bobby' may not respond positively to being called Robert. Children also have genders and getting the 'he' or 'she' correct is essential. In the mother's eyes, if you cannot even get the sex of her child right, how can she trust your treatment? It is unacceptable to talk about the child as 'it'. Words which refer to the child as a newborn, baby, infant, toddler, teenager or adolescent, are appropriate. Words such as 'your kid' and 'your offspring' are not acceptable. A kid is a young goat, while the title 'offspring' does not invoke feelings of warmth, pride or love.

Taking a good history requires experience and a sound background in paediatric knowledge. It also requires knowledge of cultural practices, and such an understanding needs to be expressed. The traditional healer may well be part of the team caring for the child. With time, it becomes easier to direct your history-taking in a particular direction, as new cues point the way forward. You should remain the listener at all times. Do not jump to premature conclusions, and allow the mother to tell her story in her own words, while taking the time to ensure mutual understanding. A word such as 'diarrhoea', for example, may have different interpretations, and further questioning will be needed to define exactly what the mother means when using a particular word or description. In history-taking, the 'listen and hear' aspect is as essential as is the 'look and see' principle in physical examination.

During history-taking it is useful to record important statements made by the mother. These are often accurate and revealing. Remember that 'right answers' require right questions in the first place, and that the way questions are structured or framed often determines the value of the answer. This is particularly important when working through an interpreter. In this situation, great care must be taken in assessing answers. The party game in which the final version of the 'story' whispered from person to person bears no relationship to the original, suggests an important lesson. Children themselves may give valuable information, and asking them directly what they feel, or where they hurt, and so on, can be useful, especially with children over the age of five. Children with chronic or recurrent ailments will often surprise you by their insight into their condition.

Remember to be culture and gender sensitive at all times.

Gaining more information

While taking a history, listen carefully to what is being said, how it is being said, and watch accompanying facial expressions, body, and hand movements. These all give information regarding the state of mind and indicate feelings such as anxiety or even guilt. The reliability of the information being obtained can thus be judged during the interview.

Do not make premature judgements. In particular, do not express surprise or dismay at the advice or management given by nurses, doctors, or traditional healers. You are hearing only one interpretation which may be incorrect or incomplete. On the other hand, it might be accurate and will then require that appropriate action be taken.

Frame your questions in non-threatening ways. Avoid direct or confrontational questions such as 'Why didn't you?' Each problem requires a specific and structured frame of questions which can provide important information. Such information may be of a positive or negative nature. The presence or absence of a particular aspect can be equally important, for example cyanosis in heart disease, severe vomiting in diarrhoea, pyrexia preceding a convulsion, or a family history of allergy in a wheezing child.

When asking questions or giving explanations, always use simple language and lay terms. Many 'standard' medical words, which are taken for granted as being easily understood, can in fact cause confusion and be misinterpreted by parents, even if they are well educated.

The parents will also have certain questions which need to be answered. These will firstly revolve around what is wrong with the child, and why or how this occurred. Next, they will want to know what is going to happen to their child, what problems can be expected, and finally, whether the problem will recur, and what can be done to stop it recurring. At the same time, it is necessary to assess their ability to cope with information and present this at an appropriate level. There may also be unspoken fears and anxieties; even if these are unfounded, they will need to be discussed and dealt with.

An assessment of the parents' ability to recognise possible complications of the present illness, to administer medication correctly, and to assess further progress will also govern management of the child. Outpatient / home management is the ideal to strive for. Admission to hospital is justified and determined by the patient's specific needs, with social circumstances also taken into account. Hospital stays should be for as short a period as possible. In general, children are safer at home than in an infective environment of a hospital, unless they require oxygen, IV fluids, IV antibiotics, nasogastric feeding, or special investigations not available to an outpatient.

Reactions to health problems

These are often fear and anxiety. Reactions differ widely and depend on age, gender, personality, and cultural, social, and economic circumstances. Even if there is no serious basis for such reactions, the doctor / nurse must be aware of their presence in the mind of the patient or parent in order to deal with any misconception or distortion. Reassurance must be given and fears relieved whenever possible. The clinician, particularly in paediatrics, must be a caring person. 'Caring for' is the secret in the 'care of' the patient.

When you have taken the full history, record the important details, both positive and negative, and then define the problem(s). This will help you to decide which system(s) must be examined particularly carefully. The history will often produce a working diagnosis, but keep an open mind until the examination has been completed.

Remember that four factors should be considered:

- Assessment of the **current problem / diagnosis** and structuring a plan for appropriate management.
- Assessment of **co-existing problems**, for example delayed development.
- Awareness of the parents' hidden or **unspoken fears** regarding the child's problem(s) and alleviating these.
- Assessment of the parent or guardian's ability to **understand** the nature of the problem, and the likelihood of their following your advice / instructions.

History-taking: Detailed

The problem-oriented medical record system (POMR) consists of:
- Basic information about the patient (the data base).
- The problem list.
- Plans for each problem.

Basic information about the patient: The data base

This consists of information about the patient derived from:
a) history-taking with reference to any existing clinical notes; b) physical examination findings; and c) routine investigations.

The history

A full history should include information about the following aspects:

- **The presenting complaint** (P/C); words of the mother / patient, etc.
- **Present history**: A full account of the present illness including the following:
  - Health prior to this illness / problem.
  - Onset.
  - Progression.
  - Accompanying signs or symptoms.
  - Contacts (if infectious illness is a possibility).
  - Current therapy (prescribed, used, tried till now).
  - Assess reliability of information being given.
- **Past history**: These aspects will vary in importance, depending on the patient's age as well as his or her current and previous problem(s). The following factors should be looked at:
  - Antenatal: Drugs, rubella, maternal disease in pregnancy, smoking, alcohol.
  - Natal (birth): Place and method of delivery, gestational age, birth weight.
  - Postnatal problems: Jaundice, incubator, length of hospital stay, other problems.
  - Feeding and nutrition: Type, quantity, strength, and frequency of feeds.
  - Growth and development: Assess growth pattern, screen for standard milestones, for example age when first sitting, walking, talking.
  - Previous illnesses: Whether related to present problem or not, especially rheumatic fever, TB, diabetes, allergy (Note: Medicines).
- **Immunisations**: BCG, DPT, Poliomyelitis, Measles, MMR, Hepatitis B, HIB, and any others.
- **Family history**: Parents, siblings, medical, and socio-economic background, including social problems, family planning, housing, and income if necessary (use tact in obtaining these facts).
- **Special questions**: These questions relate to individual systems and must concentrate on the involved or affected system(s), for example:
  - Cardiovascular (cyanosis, dyspnoea, oedema).
  - Respiratory (cough, wheeze, tachypnoea, snoring, mouth breathing, halitosis, haemoptysis, sputum).
  - Central nervous (headache, convulsions, sight, hearing, behaviour).
  - Gastrointestinal (weight – over, under, or normal for age, appetite, vomiting, diarrhoea, jaundice, bowel action, melaena, worms).

- ○ Skin (eczema, other rashes).
- ○ Urinary tract (frequency of micturition, enuresis, urine colour, blood in urine [beware of pigments resembling blood], bladder control, stream, dysuria).
- ○ Endocrine (growth, polyuria, polydypsia).
- ○ Musculo-skeletal (gait, pain, swelling).

Physical examination (See p. 8)

Routine investigations

These could include FBC, ESR, CXR, Mantoux, urine, and stool for microscopy and culture. (Not done as a routine at a primary care consultation, but could be done for a hospital admission.)

Problem list

If a definite diagnosis or problem can be defined as a result of your findings so far, record this, but do not make tentative guesses.

List all problems, which give a concise overview of the situation. Number problems individually, for example 1) Pneumonia; 2) Failure to thrive; 3) Anaemia, and so forth.

Initial plans for each problem

A plan of approach or management along the following lines must be made for each problem:

- Diagnosis (including further tests still to be done)   Dx
- Choice of therapy   Rx
- Explanation to patient / parent   Ex

Progress notes for each problem when seen at follow-up

These are written under each numbered problem-heading, and relate to that specific numbered problem, for example:

1) Pneumonia

- Subjective information S (Says)
- Objective information O (Observe i.e. during examination)
- Assessment / Interpretation A (Assess)
- Plan for future action P (Plan) Dx, Rx, Ex

Table 1.1 Progress notes

	Content	Explanation
S	Subjective information	What the person says
O	Objective information	What you observe during the examination
A	Assessment / Interpretation	Your assessment
P	Plan for future action	The plan for future action (Dx, Rx, Ex)

Physical examination

Approach

When you approach the child you must do the following:
- Make friends first: Play first – examine later.
- Work slowly and easily.
- Be friendly and gentle: Patience is essential.
- Look and see: Do not just look.
- Warm hands and instruments.

This will help the child relax and cooperate.

Position / place for examination

This varies considerably:
- Under six months: On the couch or bed.
- Six months to three or four years: Start with child on mother's lap.
- Over four years: Standing or sitting up; the child may not like lying down.

Remove the child's clothing gradually, but undress him or her fully. Toys or sweets may be used to divert attention.

Order of examination

The order of the examination is flexible. In general, look before you feel and listen before you 'hurt' or make the patient cry, that is, do upsetting and disturbing procedures last, for example examination of the ears and throat.

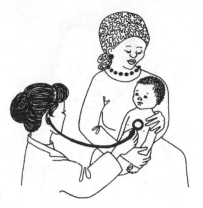

Figure 1.2 Possible position for examination

In most systems, the standard techniques of inspection, palpation, percussion, and auscultation, which cover the different aspects of clinical findings, are all required for a full assessment.

Inspection (Look and see)

This is the act of visually observing the patient, his or her general state / condition, and the many and varying aspects of each particular system, both for normality and abnormality.

Time spent on observation is time well spent.

Palpitation

This makes use of the sense of touch to assess factors such as texture, crepitance, temperature, moisture, vibration, pulsation, swelling, rigidity or spasticity, organ location and size, presence of lumps or masses, and assesses the subjective feeling of tenderness or pain by observing the reaction to palpation. Watch the facial expression.

More information can be obtained by **careful observation** than by any other single part of the examination. Each system must be fully observed before it is examined.

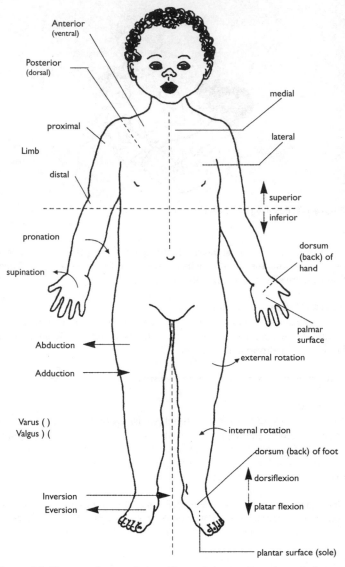

Figure 1.3 The neutral anatomical position and commonly used terminology

Percussion

This involves tapping with the middle finger of one hand on the middle finger of the other hand, which is firmly applied to the patient's body surface, in order to determine the density, location, and size of the underlying structures.

Auscultation

This assesses sounds produced in the heart, lungs, and gastrointestinal tract and checks for the presence of bruits or murmurs in the vascular system. Such sounds are best heard through a stethoscope.

Routine observations

The following must be checked in routine observations:
- Weight and percentile.
- Height and percentile.
- Weight for height.
- Head circumference (when indicated).
- Temperature: Axillary, not oral or rectal. Normal is 36,5–37 °C.
- Pulse: Rate/minute; rhythm, volume, and character – see CVS.
- Urinalysis (when indicated).
- Haemoglobin (when indicated).

Appearance
- Does this suggest some syndrome, that is, does the child look strange or dysmorphic?
- Does the child look mentally retarded / slow?
- Is he or she cooperative or not?
- Note if ill, distressed, toxic, or shocked.
- Note if well cared for or not.
- Note general nutritional status.

Skin
- Cyanosis / jaundice / pallor / oedema.
- Flushed.
- State of hydration: Look at fontanelle, eyes, skin turgor, mouth; also assess peripheral circulation / capillary filling time.
- Excoriated: Note perineal (nappy) area.
- Wasting, for example redundant skin folds especially on thighs, buttocks, and abdomen (beware of diagnosing this as dehydration).
- Purpura / bruising.

- Café au lait spots / other pigmentation / depigmentation.
- Rashes / eczema.
- Non-specific pigmented rashes (think of HIV).
- Scars.
- Skin tests, for example Mantoux / Heaf; also look for a BCG scar.

Terms used to describe lesions of the skin

Lesions of the skin are described as follows:
- **Macule**: Flat lesion; possibly erythematous, hypo- or hyperpigmented.
- **Papule**: Raised solid lesion.
- **Vesicle**: Raised lesion containing clear fluid.
- **Pustule**: Fluid in the vesicle becomes opaque due to presence or pus cells (white blood cells).
- **Bullae**: Large fluid-containing, blister-like lesions.

Types of rash

These may be erythematous or haemorrhagic.
- **Erythematous**: Will blanch on pressure, as these are due to vascular dilatation.
  o Macular: Flat.
  o Papular: Raised.
  o Morbilliform (measles-like): Both macular and papular elements.
  o Roseolar: Pink (as in roseola infantum).
  o Urticarial (allergic): Large, well-defined papules, often itchy, normal skin in-between lesions.
  o Scarlatiniform: Bright red, fine diffuse rash.
  o Vesicular / Pustular: Fluid-containing.
  o Eczematous: Often crusted and wet, or dry and scaly.
- **Purpuric or haemorrhagic**: Will not blanch on pressure, as blood is extravascular.
  o Petechiae: Pinpoint lesions.
  o Purpura: Larger, reddish-purple lesions.
  o Ecchymosis: Resembles large bruises on the skin.

Do the following to differentiate these two groups: on pressing with a finger, erythematous lesions blanch (capillary dilation) while haemorrhagic ones do not (blood is extravascular).

Secondary changes in rashes

These may occur with scaling, desquamation, staining, scarring, scabbing, or secondary infection of the skin, all of which may greatly alter

the appearance of the original rash. When describing any rash, assess the following:
- Type of rash.
- Distribution, that is, parts of body involved.
- Progression of the rash.
- How it has regressed.
- How it has healed.

Head / face
- Shape: Symmetrical / asymmetrical.
- Circumference of head: Normal, large, or small. Smaller than the third percentile (microcephaly).
- Hair: Distribution, quality, texture, lice, impetigo, or ringworm.
- Fontanelle: Open or closed? If open, is it normal, tense, or sunken? If sunken, assess hydration.
- Is there craniotabes? (Uncomfortable test, be gentle.) Not of significance if child is under three months.

Eyes
- Sunken (dehydration).
- Slant / epicanthic folds / ptosis.
- Proptosis.
- Squint.
- Conjunctivae: Purpura / jaundice / anaemia / conjunctivitis.
- Cornea: Normal or scarred.
- Are pupils of equal size and do they react equally to light?
- Is there evidence of cataract or corneal opacity?
- Vision: Do they fix on an object, follow light, etc.

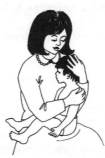

Figure 1.4 Position for examination of ear

Ears

- Note the general appearance and compare the shape, size, and situation of both ears (i.e. low set, malrotated or normal), and any other abnormalities, such as pre-auricular skin tag, sinus or bat ears.
- Examine the normal ear first and use for comparison.
- Ask and check if ear, especially tragus, is painful to touch and whether pain is experienced while chewing (as occurs in otitis externa).

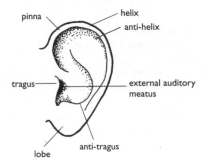

Figure 1.5 External ear anatomy

- Draw the outer part of the ear upwards and backwards in the older child, or downwards and backwards in the infant to straighten the canal.
- Note condition of the eardrum (tympanic membrane): May be normal, inflamed, bulging, retracted or perforated. Normal drums are whitish / pink and glisten, but this changes with disease. Distinguish the eardrum from the inner end of the auditory canal by the handle of the malleus, which runs downward and is attached behind the drum.
- Assessment of hearing can be done now or during CNS examination.

An auriscope is used for the examination of both the auditory canal and the drum.

Difficulty in seeing the tympanic membrane may be due to:
- Poor technique.
- Wax, foreign body or discharge in auditory canal.
- Dirty auriscope lens / weak batteries.
- Faulty setting of the light bulb.
- A tympanic membrane which is more horizontal than usual.

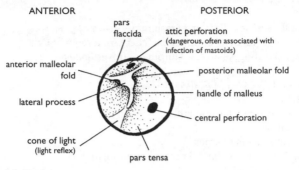

Figure 1.6 Eardrum

Table 1.2 Causes of eardrum abnormalities

Finding	Interpretation	Examples
Bright red drum Blood vessels visible on drum	Inflammation	Acute middle ear infection (otitis media)
Absent light reflex	Bulging of drum and inflammation	Acute otitis media
Yellowish drum	Pus or serum behind drum	Acute or chronic otitis media
Bubbles behind drum	Serous fluid in middle ear	Chronic serous otitis media
Absent or diminished landmarks	Thickening of drum	Chronic otitis media or otitis externa
Oval dark areas	Perforation	Recent or old rupture of drum
Malleus very prominent	Retraction of drum	Obstruction of Eustachian tube
Bluish drum	Blood behind drum	Skull fracture

Nose
- Alar flare of nostrils (sign of respiratory distress).
- Discharge: Bilateral or unilateral (check for foreign body).
- Large pale boggy (swollen) turbinates (investigate allergy).

Mouth, teeth, and pharynx
- Halitosis.
- Cheilosis / angular stomatitis.
- Dental caries.
- Thrush / ulcers / herpes.
- Koplik's spots: On buccal mucosa opposite molars.
- High arched palate.
- Cleft lip or palate (**Note**: Posterior uvula cleft often missed).

Tongue
- Tongue-tie: Can tongue reach back of teeth?
- Geographical tongue: Of interest but of no significance.

Throat and tonsils
Examine these last, as this often upsets the child:
- Inflamed, follicles.
- Membrane.
- Post-nasal drip.
- Hoarse voice.
- Snoring / stridor.

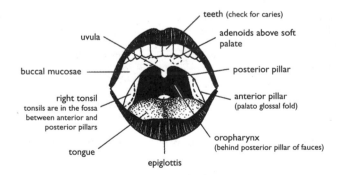

Figure 1.7 Mouth and oropharynx

Lymph nodes

Determine the following when you examine the lymph nodes:
- Site / location.
- Size.
- Tenderness.
- Consistency.

Generalised, painless enlargement often a marker of HIV.

Main areas

Examine the following areas:
- Head and neck: Specific groups of lymph nodes (see Figure 1.8).
- Axillary.
- Inguinal.
- Groups of glands may enlarge secondary to infection in their drainage areas.

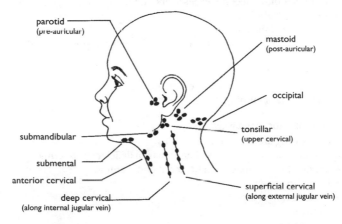

Figure 1.8 Lymph nodes (Head and neck)

Wrist / hands / nails

- Rickets (thickening of distal ends of radius and ulna).
- Palmar erythema: After puberty, sign of severe liver disease.
- Single crease: Simian crease (normal or syndrome, e.g. Down syndrome).
- Syndactyly (fused digits); polydactyly (extra digits).

- Clubbing of fingers secondary to:
  - Chronic suppurative lung disease, for example bronchiectasis or lung abscess.
  - Cyanotic congenital heart disease.
  - Bacterial endocarditis.
  - Chronic liver disease: Cirrhosis.
  - Chronic diarrhoeal conditions, for example Crohn's disease or ulcerative colitis.
  - Multiple parasites. (**Note**: Trichuris [Whipworm])
  - Familial: Look at parent's nails.

Clubbing

There are three degrees of clubbing:
- Mild clubbing:
  - Loss of normal nail / cuticle angle.
  - Nail base also becomes soft, shiny, and spongy.
  - Cuticles often become excessively friable.
- Moderate clubbing:
  - Beaking of the nail.
  - Increase in the pulp of the finger in the anterior-posterior (AP) diameter.
- Severe clubbing:
  - Increase in the transverse diameter.
  - Drumstick clubbing.

Other nail abnormalities

The following are other abnormalities:
- Koilonychia: Spoon-shaped nails in iron deficiency anaemia.
- Splinter haemorrhages: In bacterial endocarditis.
- Pallor (in anaemia).
- Chronic fungal infection.
- Cyanosis.
- Nail-biting.

Genitalia

Male

- Penis: Check for hypospadias / phimosis / abnormally large or small size.
- Testicles: Are they in scrotum, or can they be brought down into the scrotum? (Check for undescended testes.)

- Hernial sites: Check that these are intact.
- Urine voiding: Strength of stream.

Female
- Clitoris: Is it unusually large? (masculinisation)
- Check labia for fusion (intersex).
- Check vagina for discharge and note its character (whether bloody, purulent or mucoid).
- Hernial sites: Check that these are intact.

Spine
This examination depends on the age of the child:
- **Infant**: Assess for spinal defects especially lower end (sacral dimple, sinus, tuft of hair, or fluid-filled swelling). Coccygeal dimple or sinus is normal.
- **Children**: Assess for scoliosis (with child standing, look from behind).

Legs and feet
There are three aspects to look at:
- Bow-legs, knock-knees or leg shortening.
- Flat or club feet.
- Asymmetrical skin creases of infant's thighs (check for congenital dislocation of hip).

Respiratory system
Important points found on general examination:
- Tachypnoea.
- Alar flare.
- Recession. } The five important signs indicating respiratory distress
- Grunting.
- Cyanosis.
- Pulse rate.
- Clubbing (bronchiectasis, lung abscess, chronic HIV).
- Anaemia (aggravates associated hypoxia).
- Sitting upright (not wanting to lie down).
- Use of accessory muscles.
- Restlessness or anxiety.
- Orthopnoea.
- Cough – type and timing (see Table 1.3).

Table 1.3 Type and timing of cough

Cough	Suggests
Croupy	Barking associated with stridor
Chesty	Moist, fruity, productive
Non-productive, nocturnal	Post-nasal drip, asthma
Paroxysmal	Pertussis, foreign body
Bovine, brassy	Tracheitis
On exercise	Asthma
During or after a feed	Incoordination of swallowing Reflux / aspiration
Productive in morning	Cystic fibrosis, asthma
Absence during sleep	Psychogenic

Inspection

Note: Most respiratory pathology can be assessed or detected by careful observation. Stand back and observe!

Shape of the chest
- Normal.
- Barrel (increased anterior-posterior diameter): Air trapping.
- Pectus excavatum (funnel chest).
- Pectus carinatum (pigeon chest).
- Harrison's sulcus (rickets): Normal diaphragm pulls on soft ribs.
- Chronic lung disease sulcus (at insertion of diaphragm): Due to increased pull on normal ribs.
- Symmetry: Are the right and left sides equal, or is there bulging or flattening of one side?

Movement of the chest
- Rate of respiration: Normal, increased or decreased. Respiratory rate must be taken for a full minute.

Table 1.4 Normal range of respiratory rate

Age	Respiratory rate/minute
Newborn	40–60
Infant	25–35
12 months	25–30
4th year	25
8th year	14–20
15th year	12–15

- Pattern of respiration:
  - Normal.
  - Prolonged inspiration (upper airway obstruction).
  - Prolonged expiration (lower airway obstruction, e.g. bronchospasm / wheezing).
  - Grunting (breathing out against a closed glottis); common in hyaline membrane disease or pneumonia in young children.
- Rhythm of respiration:
  - Periodic, for example in preterm.
  - Cheyne Stokes (terminal pattern of respiration, dependent on CO_2 drive).
  - Acidotic (Kussmaul): Deep and sighing (may be rapid in infants).
  - Shallow / painful (pleuritic – uncommon in children).
- Asymmetry of movement (remember air entry gives rise to chest movement) from underlying:
  - Effusion, exudate (pus), transudate (clear fluid) or blood.
  - Collapse / consolidation.
  - Pneumothorax.
  - Fibrosis / destruction of lung substance.
- Recession on respiration:
  - Due to increased effort of inspiration; the greater intra-thoracic negative pressure created draws in the soft tissues, as lungs are either stiffer than normal (e.g. pneumonia), or there is obstruction to air flowing in (as occurs in stridor).
  - May be:
    - Supraclavicular (above clavicle).
    - Suprasternal (above sternum).
    - Substernal (below sternum in epigastrium).

- Sternal (sternum itself): Soft in children.
- Intercostal (between ribs).
- Subcostal (below rib margin).

Palpation

- To determine expansion: The two-handed technique to assess the degree and symmetry of chest movement is of some use only in older, cooperative children. Inspection is far more accurate, especially in young children.
  - Do right and left sides of the chest move equally?
- Vocal fremitus (feeling the vibration of the voice with the flat of the hand on the chest wall).
  - Normal.
  - Increased over collapse and consolidation (better conduction to the surface).
  - Decreased with pneumothorax or effusion.
- Heart apex (pushed or pulled) away from normal position: Mediastinal shift.
- Position of trachea in suprasternal notch (difficult to assess and often inaccurate in small children).

Percussion

With percussion, sensation of resonance or lack thereof is as important as the actual note created.

- Percuss from resonant to less resonant areas.
- Have long axis of finger parallel to ribs or edge of organ, for example upper border of liver.
- Keep finger in close contact with chest wall.
- Compare right and left equivalent areas both anteriorly and posteriorly.
- Determine upper border of the liver (normal is fourth to fifth right intercostal space in the mid-clavicular line).
- Normal resonance.
- Increased resonance:
  - Pneumothorax.
  - Air trapping, for example bronchospasm / bronchiolitis / emphysema.
- Decreased resonance:
  - Consolidation, that is, not air-filled lung.
  - Pleural thickening.
  - Fibrosis / collapse of lung.

- Stony / dull:
  ○ Fluid / pus / blood.

Auscultation

Character of breath sounds:

- **Normal breath sounds**:
  Caused by turbulence of air flowing through the larynx and in the larger airways.
- **Vesicular breath sounds**:
  This describes the quality of normal breath sounds. Breath sounds in children are generally harsher (broncho-vesicular) than in adults. This is especially so over the right upper lobe (RUL), because of the thin chest wall, relatively large airways, and their proximity to the chest surface.
- **Tracheal breath sounds**:
  This breath sound, where both the inspiratory and expiratory elements have a harsh, superficial quality, is normally heard when listening over the trachea with a stethoscope.
- **Bronchial breathing**.
  When 'tracheal breath sounds' are heard over other areas of the chest (i.e. not over the trachea), it is called bronchial breathing and indicates consolidation of the lung. The consolidated areas conduct breath sounds to the surface better than normal air-filled lungs, thus they sound harsher and the expiratory component is emphasised.
- **Decreased breath sounds**:
  These do not necessarily indicate decreased air entry, as an effusion or pleural thickening may damp down breath sounds while air entry into the lung is still occurring reasonably normally. Observing chest movement and comparing the right and left sides best assess air entry.

Vocal resonance (Voice sound heard through a stethoscope)

Patient says 'one, one, one' or 'ninety-nine' or just cries.

- Normal.
- Increased (over area of consolidation and / or collapse).
- Decreased (overlying effusion, pneumothorax).

Added sounds

Note: Always compare equivalent areas on right and left sides of the chest both anteriorly and posteriorly.

- **Grunting**: Patient breathes out against a closed glottis. This increases intralumenal pressure in the lungs and small airways on expiration to help prevent their collapse, and also improves oxygen transfer. Occurs in pneumonia and respiratory distress syndrome, for example hyaline membrane disease.
- **Wheezing**: A long, 'whistling', dry, continuous sound, which may be audible with the ear or through a stethoscope. Usually predominantly an expiratory sound, but may have an inspiratory component when obstruction is severe. Caused by lower airways obstruction, which may be due to bronchospasm, oedema, secretions or any obstruction in the lumen, wall, or outside the wall (such as compressing lymph nodes).
- **Crackles**: Crackling, wet, discontinuous sounds, fine or coarse; mainly inspiratory short sounds. Caused by opening of the small bronchioli with sticky fluid in them. Occur in parenchymal disease, for example pneumonia, pulmonary oedema, etc. Crackles are fine (small airways) or coarse (larger airways).
- **Stridor**: A harsh, crowing, vibratory, predominantly inspiratory sound; due to obstruction of the upper extrathoracic airway. If there is an expiratory element as well, this means severe narrowing: danger sign!
- **Friction rub (pleural)**: Sounds like a crackling tissue paper. Due to inflamed surfaces rubbing on each other. Occurs in both inspiration and expiration. An uncommon sign in children.

Cardiovascular system

Important points found on general examination:

Poor weight gain

Cyanosis

Oxygenated haemoglobin is pink, but when deoxygenated, it turns blue. In the presence of severe anaemia, cyanosis is more difficult to detect clinically because of the low haemoglobin.

Peripheral cyanosis

- Due to cold extremities or poor peripheral circulation.
- Local obstruction of the circulation.
- As a result, stagnant blood in the peripheral areas has oxygen removed from it by the tissues; these areas then look blue.

Central cyanosis
All the circulating blood is blue, and therefore extremities, tongue, and mucous membranes are blue.

Causes:
- **Respiratory (decreased oxygenation)**: Severe lung pathology, for example pneumonia.
- **Cardiac**: Right to left shunt in heart, for example in congenital heart disease: Fallot's tetralogy, or a common mixing situation.

Erythema marginatum / nodules / arthritis
Investigate for rheumatic fever.

Oedema
- Generalised / dependent (although it may occur, it is a late and therefore poor sign of cardiac failure in children).
- Localised: Not of cardiac origin.

Nails
- Clubbing: Bacterial endocarditis (SBE), cyanotic congenital heart disease.
- Splinter haemorrhages (SBE).

Tachypnoea or dyspnoea or sweating
This is an important sign and may indicate underlying cardiac failure.

Anaemia
Aggravates cardiac condition or polycythaemia (congenital cyanotic heart disease).

Pulse
The following aspects are important:
- **Rate**: Check rate and note whether normal, increased or decreased. If febrile, each 1 °C rise in temperature above normal increases pulse rate by approximately ten beats per minute.

Table 1.5 Normal range

Age	Beats per minute
Birth–3 months	120–160
1 year	80–140
2 years	80–130
3 years	80–120
Older	70–115

- **Rhythm**: Regular or irregular. Sinus arrhythmia is an increased rate on inspiration and slowing on expiration (normal physiological event).
- **Volume**: Small (thready / weak), normal, or full.
- **Character**:
  - Collapsing pulse (water hammer pulse) occurs in aortic incompetence, patent ductus arteriosus, and AV fistulae due to pressure run-off. High systolic pressure with low or absent diastolic pressure.
  - Pulsus paradoxus: Decreased volume (pressure) of pulse on inspiration. Occurs in constrictive pericarditis, severe asthma, and severe stridor.
  - Feel for weak or absent femoral pulses (coarctation of the aorta). Radio-femoral delay – difficult in small childen with rapid pulse rate.
- Capillary filling time:
  - Check capillary filling time (normal 4 seconds) and peripheral perfusion.

Blood pressure

Width of blood pressure cuff should be two-thirds the length of the upper arm (cubital fossa to axillary skin fold). If cuff is too large, false low reading will result.

- Estimated by:
  - Palpation (systolic only).
  - Oscillation of needle or upper border of mercury (systolic only).
  - Auscultation (systolic and diastolic): Systolic: where sound is first heard; diastolic: where it softens (not where it disappears).

Table 1.6 Normal upper limits at different ages (in millimetres of mercury)

Years	Systolic	Diastolic
0–3	110	65
3–7	120	70
7–10	130	75
10–13	140	80

Anatomy

The apex beat of the heart is the lowermost, outermost point at which cardiac pulsation is maximally felt during systole.

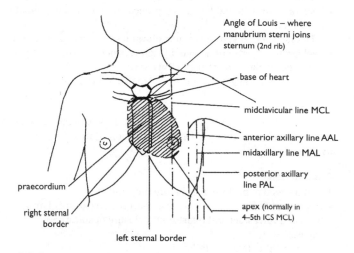

Figure 1.9 Anatomy and reference points

Examination of the heart

Inspection

- Shape of thorax: Bulge over praecordium or asymmetry of chest indicates long-standing cardiomegaly.
- Look for signs of raised jugular venous pressure (JVP). Patient at 45°, measure height in centimetres above angle of Louis. A raised JVP

occurs in cardiac failure. (Cannot be assessed in a crying or screaming child.)
- Active praecordium / pulsations.
- Apex beat position often visible.

Palpation
- Apex beat:
  - Normally found in the fourth to fifth left intercostal space, MCL (first find it and then determine its position).
  - May be displaced, to right or left and down. Cause: pulled or pushed by lung pathology or cardiomegaly. In mediastinal shift situations, for example large one-sided pleural effusion, heart is also displaced.
  - May be impalpable. Fluid round heart as in pericarditis or fat chest wall.
- Feel for thrills with flat hand over praecordium (check for palpable murmurs).
  - Define whether systolic or diastolic and site of maximum intensity.
- Feel for increased cardiac activity, left ventricular hypertrophy (LVH), right ventricular hypertrophy (RVH).
- Feel for hepatomegaly (important sign of cardiac failure).

Percussion
This is used to define the size of the heart. It is difficult and inaccurate unless heart is markedly enlarged. Percussion is, therefore, often of little use in children.

Auscultation
This may need to be done first before the child cries.
- Heart sounds (valve closure): First heart sound closure of mitral and tricuspid valves, second heart sound closure of aortic and pulmonary valves.
- Gallop rhythm (cardiac failure).
- Murmurs: Systolic or diastolic (see Chapter 5); site of maximum intensity and radiation.

Gastrointestinal system
Important points found on general examination:
- Nutritional state / physical growth / percentile chart.
- State of hydration.
- Presence of oedema (establish whether nutritional or hepatic).

- Presence of clubbing (cirrhosis, ulcerative colitis, Crohn's disease, multiple parasites).
- White nails (hypoalbuminaemia).
- Jaundice.
- Liver palms (pink) usually only after puberty (hormonal effect), signs of liver failure, altered level of consciousness (hepatic coma).
- Presence of pallor due to anaemia (check for GIT blood loss, iron deficiency).

Examination of abdomen

Anatomical areas serve to:
- Divide the abdomen for descriptive purposes.

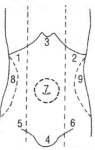

1. Right hypochondrium
2. Left hypochondrium
3. Epigastrium
4. Hypogastrium
5. Right iliac fossa
6. Left iliac fossa
7. Periumbilical
8. Right lumbar (posterior)
9. Left lumbar (posterior)

Figure 1.10 Anatomical areas: terminology

- Locate site of pain / mass / organ, etc.

Inspection

Shape

- Scaphoid. In newborn, this may indicate a diaphragmatic hernia.
- Distension or fullness: Cause may be:
  - Fluid (ascites).
  - Flatus (gas).
  - Faeces.
  - Fat.
  - Food.
  - Enlarged organ/s.
  - Mass.
  - Fetus in menarchial girls.

The most common causes are flatus and fluid.

Respiratory abdominal movement

This may be affected in conditions involving the diaphragm, especially if asymmetrical or paradoxical. Also poor movement in severe abdominal distension from whatever cause. With inspiration, abdomen normally moves outward, but with diaphragmatic paralysis it moves inwards.

Umbilicus

- Everted or 'smiling' (may be associated with ascites).
- Hernia (note diameter of defect in cm).
- Septic (in newborn).

Hernial sites

- Inguinal (assess with patient standing or sitting up to increase intra-abdominal pressure).
- Umbilical.
- Supra- or periumbilical.

Visible peristalsis

Is this because the child is very thin, or is it due to early intestinal obstruction?

Distended veins on abdomen (flowing upwards)

These may indicate portal hypertension or inferior vena caval obstruction.

Palpation

To determine the presence and nature of pain, tenderness, abdominal organs, and any masses.

The patient must be relaxed and the examiner's hand warm. Use flat hand and radial border of index finger. Watch the facial expression for signs of pain while doing a gentle, general palpation. Palpation must be light. Deep palpation is only done when feeling the kidneys.

- Guarding is a voluntary protective muscular contraction.
- Rigidity is involuntary and may be generalised or localised.
- Tenderness: Direct or rebound? (peritoneal irritation)
- Single hand palpation for other organs / masses.
- Bimanual palpation for kidneys.

Percussion

- If distended, resonant (gas) or dull (fluid)?
- If ascites (free fluid) is present, there may be a fluid thrill. This is

detected by feeling the thrill conducted through the ascitic fluid after tapping sharply on the other side of the abdomen (with a helper's hand held on the abdomen to stop conduction through the abdominal wall).

- Shifting dullness: Shown by the level of percussed dullness changing when the patient is turned from lying on their back and placed on their side. Level of dullness rises on the side nearest the bed.
- Percuss above the pubis for bladder dullness (if distended / full).

Auscultation

If necessary, listen for at least a few minutes.
Bowel sounds (borborygmi):

- Normal.
- Increased (in diarrhoea, or for mechanical reasons, e.g. early on in obstruction).
- Decreased.
- Silent (absent): May be ileus.

Rectal examination

Not done as a routine in children, as it is uncomfortable and embarrassing. The following indications are important:

- Bleeding per rectum, discomfort on stooling, fissure.
- Diagnostic (checking for loose stools to account for clinical dehydration).
- Constipation (checking for impacted rectal faecal mass).
- Soiling (impacted faeces are hard, while in faecal loading faeces in rectum are often soft).

Anus must be examined in all newborn babies for presence or absence. Blood on stools may be due to an anal fissure or low rectal polyp.

Examination of vomitus

Features

- Copious / projectile / frothy and sour-smelling (check for pyloric stenosis).
- Effortless and following feeds (check for gastro-oesophageal reflux).

Content

- Food / medicine / toxin: Keep if poisoning suspected.
- Blood:

- o Fresh (bright red).
- o Clots (large bleed).
- o Old (black or brown in colour or 'coffee-grounds').
- Bile: Green vomitus must be considered as a surgical (i.e. obstructive) cause until proven otherwise.
- Feculent: Due to low intestinal obstruction, a late ominous sign.

Examination of faeces
Colour
- Marked normal variation in colour and form, especially during neonatal period (depends on type of feed).
- Normal range: Yellow to brown / green, very soft to quite firm.
- Green: May be normal, soya bean milk feed or diarrhoea, phototherapy.
- Grey / black: Liquorice / charcoal / iron ingestion.
- Melaena (black, smelly, and sticky): Blood from nose, oesophagus or proximal bowel (high bleed), partial digestion.
- Pale: Obstructive jaundice or increased fat in steatorrhoea (malabsorption).
- Pink / other colour: Medications, for example Solphyllin®, pen V. etc.

Form and content
- Normal.
- Constipated.
- Increased fluid in diarrhoea.
- Pus cells found in dysentery or colitis.
- Slimy, contains mucus: Large bowel in origin.
- Blood: Site of possible origin:
  - o Black / melaena (very unpleasant smelling): Bleed high up.
  - o Red currant jelly (mucus and blood): Intussusception.
  - o Well mixed: Small bowel / beginning of large bowel.
  - o Poorly mixed: Lower part of colon.
  - o Stool streaked on outside only: Anus / rectum (fissure or polyp).

Abdominal organs
Liver
This lies in the right upper quadrant.

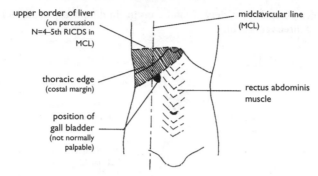

Figure 1.11 Examination of liver

Palpation

- Feel for lower edge (flat hand using radial border of index finger).
- If liver is palpable, percuss and determine position of upper border, as liver may be pushed down (air trapping in lung) and not actually enlarged.
- Take note of the following:
  ○ **Size**: Measure (in cm) from costal margin to liver edge in the mid-clavicular line.
  ○ **Edge**: Is it regular?
  ○ **Surface**: Smooth or uneven?
  ○ **Consistency**: Soft, firm or hard?
  ○ **Tenderness**: Generalised or localised?

Characteristics of a normal liver

- May normally be palpable up to 3 cm until five years of age and 1–2 cm until ten years. Of normal consistency and shape, with no tenderness.
- Moves early with respiration; down on inspiration and up with expiration, as it moves with diaphragm to which it is attached.
- Cannot be held down on expiration.
- Has two lobes with a notch between them.

Spleen

Characteristics

- Very superficial.
- Enlarges downwards and often towards left iliac fossa in children, or towards right iliac fossa as in adults. Often more laterally and posteriorly placed. Normally not palpable, but small enlargements of

spleen found in a variety of conditions in childhood, especially during first three years of life.

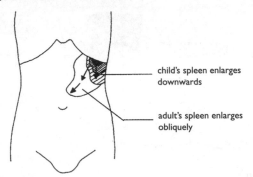

child's spleen enlarges downwards

adult's spleen enlarges obliquely

Figure 1.12 Examination of spleen

- Moves early with respiration.
- Has a medial palpable splenic notch (if sufficiently enlarged).
- Size given in cm. Measured from costal margin to tip of spleen in its longest axis (no specific reference point, as may appear anywhere along the costal margin).

Kidneys
Characteristics
- Move late with respiration, that is, late in inspiration when diaphragm eventually pushes them down.
- Bimanually palpable.
- Lobular shape; normal to feel kidneys in newborn period. At all other times, consider as abnormal if palpable.
- No medial notch.
- Fingers may be passed above upper edge (unlike spleen).

Bladder
Rises from pelvis as a suprapubic mass; seen, felt or percussed.

Other masses
See swelling / masses and method of evaluation (pp. 38–39).
Faeces may mimic a mass in many different areas.

Central nervous system

General

- Development milestones: Are these correct for age?
- Appearance of child, appropriate behaviour, intelligence.
- State of consciousness:
  - Awake, alert, and orientated.
  - Awake but confused.
  - Drowsy but fully rousable.
  - Stupor:
    - Light: Responds to superficial stimuli.
    - Deep: Responds to painful stimuli only.
  - Coma: No response to any external stimuli.

Basic assessment of some important cranial nerves

Eyes (cranial nerves two, three, four, and six):
- Can patient see?
- Is there a squint? If so:
  - Is it of long standing?
  - Recent onset (refer immediately).
- Are eye movements normal in all directions?
- Are pupils regular and do they react to light?

Face (cranial nerve seven):
- Is there any facial asymmetry while smiling or crying?

Hearing (cranial nerve eight):
- Can normal and whispered speech be heard?

Drinking / swallowing / speech (cranial nerves nine and ten):
- Normal.
- Abnormal.

Movement and tone of limbs (Motor system)

- Inspection:
  - Is there any wasting or asymmetry?
- Movement:
  - Normal: Right and left correspond and move equally in bed / cot.
- Gait:
  - Is this normal? If the child cannot walk yet, are all limbs moving equally and normally?

- Tone:
  - Increased (spastic): Check for upper motor neurone lesion.
- Tendon reflexes – compare right and left sides.
  - Increased in upper motor neurone lesion, for example cerebral palsy.
  - Decreased (hypotonic / floppy): Check for lower motor neurone lesion.

Sensory system
Very difficult to assess accurately in children. Do not use pins or needles. Use a split wooden tongue depressor as the 'sharp' instrument.

Assess for signs of meningeal irritation
- Neck stiffness or rigidity.
- Kernig's sign: Patient supine with hip flexed to 90°; pain and inability to fully extend the knee is positive; negative if can fully extend knee.
- Brudzinski sign: On flexion of neck, involuntary flexion of legs at the knees and hips is positive; negative if legs do not flex.
- Meningism: Here neck stiffness is secondary to upper respiratory tract infection or pneumonia, and not due to meningitis (exercise caution in reaching this conclusion).

Assess for signs of increased (raised) intracranial pressure
- Altered level of consciousness.
- Full fontanelle (in infants less than 18 months).
- Vomiting.
- High-pitched cry.
- Irritability.
- Headache.
- Bradycardia.
- Hypertension.

Any other abnormalities noted?

Musculoskeletal system
General approach
Inspection
- Area must be fully exposed and examined in a good light; both sides are important. Use normal side for comparison.

- Bones: Alignment / deformity / shortening.
- Soft tissues: Swelling / wasting / asymmetry.
- Skin: Colour / texture / erythema / cyanosis / pigmentation, etc.
- Scars / sinuses:
  - Are these from surgery or injury?
  - Is there suppuration?
- Prosthesis, for example calipers, special shoes (built-up, wedged).

Palpation

- Overlying skin temperature: Use flat hand and compare right and left sides.
- Local tenderness: Exact site must be mapped out.
- Soft tissues: Describe local swelling.
- Bones: Any thickening or deformity.

Joints

Determine pain or swelling. If swollen, check whether fluid or soft tissue.

Movement

- What is the range of active movement? (normal or limited)
- What is the range of passive movement? (normal or limited)
- Is movement painful?
- Is movement accompanied by crepitus?
- Fixed deformity: This exists when the joint cannot be placed in the neutral anatomical position.
- Stability of joint: Is there abnormal movement or laxity of joint ligaments?

State of peripheral circulation

Particularly important after trauma or fracture, and when limb is in plaster of Paris.

Referred symptoms: Examination as to possible sources

Table 1.7 Referred symptoms

Site of pain	Referred from (i.e. pathology in)
Shoulder	Neck or diaphragm
Knee	Hip
Jaw	Ear
Thigh	Spine
	Pelvis
	Abdomen
	Genito-urinary tract

Full general physical examination (when assessing musculoskeletal system)

This is especially important because of a wide spectrum of presentations of many conditions, for example rheumatic fever.

General approach to pain

- Site of the pain: Where does it occur?
- Duration: How long has it been there?
- Character and intensity: Type and degree.
- Periodicity: Constant or comes and goes.
- Radiation: One place or goes elsewhere.
- Aggravating factors: What makes it worse?
- Relieving factors: What makes it better?
- Associated symptoms: May be related or not.

Approach to any swelling or mass

History

- Duration (how long has it been there?)
- Onset (gradual or sudden).
- Development / progression (same, smaller, larger).

- Pain associated or not.
- Any other swellings.
- Any other symptoms of note.

Using skills of
- Inspection.
- Palpation.
- Percussion.
- Auscultation.
- Transillumination.
- Measurement.

You want to know (9 S's)
- Situation / site.
- Size.
- Shape.
- Sensitivity / sore.
- Solid / consistency.
- Surface: Ulcer, etc.
- Specific relations:
  ○ Overlying tissue / skin.
  ○ Muscle, bone, joint, nerve, and blood vessels.
- Single / multiple.
- Signs of spread: Local or general.

Diagnosis
- Anatomical: First of all, what tissue or organ is involved?
- General pathological: What process is involved? (e.g. tumour, inflammatory)
- Specific pathology: Histology / type.

Presentation of history and examination findings

Name, age, race (when medically relevant), sex, and percentile (weight / age).

History
- Presenting complaint.
- Present history.
- Past history, etc.

General examination
- 'Lay' description of condition in general terms, including nutritional state (paint verbal picture).
- Temperature.
- Appearance of head / hair / ears / eyes / nose.
- Presence or absence of lymph glands (occipital / cervical / axillary / inguinal).
- Anaemia.
- Cyanosis (central or peripheral).
- Jaundice.
- Clubbing.
- Oedema.
- Hydration (fontanelle / eyes / mouth / skin turgor and peripheral circulation).
- Skin (scars / rashes / naevi, etc.).

Next, present the abnormal or involved system first (i.e. not necessarily in the following order):

Ear, nose, and throat (ENT)
- Mouth (ulcers / thrush, etc.).
- Tonsils.
- Pharynx.
- Ears.

Respiratory system
- Rate of respiration.
- Alar flare.
- Recession.
- Cyanosis.
- Grunting.
- Pattern of respiration (prolonged inspiration or expiration).
- Percussion (normal / resonant / dull / stony dull / hyper-resonant).

- Breath sounds (normal / wheezing / crackles / bronchial breathing / stridor).

Cardiovascular system (CVS)
- Pulse rate.
- Pulses present (radical, brachial / femoral).
- Blood pressure.
- Jugular venous pressure (JVP).
- Apex beat position.
- Any thrill felt on palpation of praecordium.
- Heart sounds.
- Gallop rhythm.
- Murmurs.

Gastrointestinal system (GIT)
- Distension.
- Veins on surface.
- Umbilicus (infection / hernia).
- Tenderness / rigidity / guarding.
- Masses.
- Liver, spleen, kidneys, ascites.
- Bowel sounds.
- Genitalia / hernial sites.
- Anus.

Central nervous system (CNS)
- Appearance and behaviour.
- Level of consciousness.
- Stage of development (e.g. sitting / walking / talking, etc.).
- Vision.
- Hearing.
- Speech.
- Are all four limbs moving equally, or is gait normal?
- Is tone normal, increased or decreased?
- Neck stiffness.
- Kernig's or Brudzinski signs positive or negative?
- Is fontanelle normal, full or depressed? (infants under 18 months of age)
- Signs of raised intracranial pressure.

In summary: Very briefly summarise both relative positive and negative findings.

Define problems in order of significance: 1; 2; 3. etc.

Plan further investigation (when indicated) and the management of each problem that has been identified.

Physical growth and development

Growth

If a variety of measurements such as weight, length or head circumference are assessed in a large number of normal children, a **normal bell-shaped distribution curve** is found (see Figure 2.1). The measurements are distributed symmetrically on each side of the mean, with a larger cluster around the mean. Such a typical normal distribution curve, also called a Gaucian curve, can also be presented as a percentile chart. Fifty per cent (50%) will fall below and 50% above the mean. The mean is also called the median or standard value.

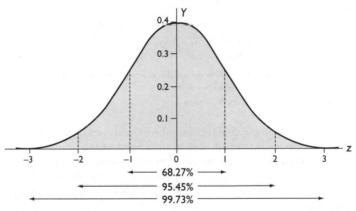

Figure 2.1 Normal distribution curve

Percentiles

Definition: A specific point in a distribution curve which has a given percentage of cases above and below it. The 50th percentile is seen as the midpoint of a normal distribution curve with 50% of cases below it.

The lower limit of normal is taken for practical purposes as the third percentile and the upper limit as the 97th percentile. Only 3% of normal cases fall below the third percentile and 3% above the 97th percentile. Some charts use the 5th and 95th percentiles.

A normal distribution pattern for weight, length, and head circumference has been established for every month of age in the first two years of life, and for every two months until the age of 12 years. This was done by measuring hundreds of normal children in each age group.

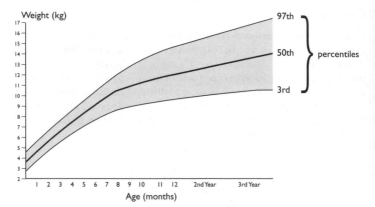

The shaded area represents the whole normal distribution range. Some percentile charts use the 5th and 95th percentiles as the normal range.

Figure 2.2 Normal distribution range

From such a range of normal measurements, percentile charts have been drawn up for weight, length, and head circumference. These are often named according to where the measurements were done, for example Boston.

Weight

The most rapid period of growth after the intrauterine period is during the first two years of life, especially during the first year.

Average birth weight is doubled by five months and trebled by one year. Ideally, the weight of every child seen at a clinic or hospital should be plotted on a percentile chart, rather than trying to rely on memory as a guide. If no percentile charts are available, the formula given in Table 2.1 can be used to determine an average expected weight for age in years. However, it might not necessarily be applicable to the specific child.

Table 2.1 Average weight

Age	kg
Birth	3,5
5–6 months	7
I year	10
2 years	12,5
3 years	15
4–10 years	(Age × 2) + 8 (e.g. 5 years = 18 kg)

Length / height

Length is measured while the child is lying down and height is measured when the child is standing. They are both plotted on the same chart.

Length follows a similar pattern to weight. After the age of four years, the formula 100 cm plus 6 cm per year of age over four years can be used to calculate an average length.

Table 2.2 Average length (Height)

Age	cm
Birth	50
6 months	65
I year	75
2 years	87
3 years	95
4 years	100
4–10 years	100 + 6 cm per year over 4

Head circumference

Head circumference is of critical importance, as increase in head size is almost entirely dependent on ongoing brain growth (with hydrocephalus the obvious exception).

The most rapid period of brain growth is before birth and during the first and the beginning of the second year of life. More brain growth occurs during the first year after birth than in the total period from one year of age until adulthood. Most of this growth takes place during the first six months of life.

If severe nutritional insult or prolonged illness occurs during this vulnerable period, 'catch up' brain growth may be insufficient for the individual to achieve his or her full potential.

Table 2.3 Average head circumference

Age	cm
Birth	35
3 months	40
6 months	44
I year	47
2 years	50
5 years	52
Adult	56±

Physical growth

Growth depends on a number of variable factors, the two most important being genetic and environmental factors. This is why we are not all the same size or shape.

Genetic *(Hereditary)*

This refers to the type of body build inherited from the parents. If both parents are small and short, the children are likely to be small, whereas tall parents tend to have tall children. This is, however, not always the case; there are exceptions to this rule.

Environment

This includes our surroundings and the factors that influence our life and growth. The more important ones are: nutrition and health.

A diet which is incorrect in quantity or quality prevents normal growth. This can be detected on properly completed growth charts. Poor health includes specific infections, as well as serious disturbances of physiological function, such as underlying heart disease or severe congenital abnormalities. If any of the vital organs do not work properly, the child cannot grow normally.

Health and nutrition, in turn, influence each other, that is, the unhealthy child may become malnourished and the poorly nourished child then suffers more frequent infections. A serious cycle is set in motion with the one factor aggravating the other.

Percentile growth charts

These are graphs used to record a child's growth and physical development over a period of time. In these graphs one factor is plotted against another different but related factor, for example weight and age. Repeated observations are recorded at intervals.

Increasing age in a child should be accompanied by an increase in weight. The graph shows not only this, but also the rate at which it is occurring. Increase in weight by itself is not enough, as the time over which it occurred must also be taken into account.

Explanation of graph (Figure 2.3)

When seen at two months, the baby is found to weigh 4 kg.

By following a straight line up from two months and across from 4 kg, a point is plotted.

At the age of four months, the baby now weighs 5 kg, and at six months, 6 kg. These points can be joined by a line creating a graph indicating the baby's growth pattern. In a similar way, height or head circumference can be plotted.

Human beings of any given age are not all the same size, even though they may be perfectly normal and healthy. Therefore, it cannot be said that a normal newborn should weigh, for example, 3,5 kg. There is always a range of normal, in this case from 2,5 to 4,0 kg.

It is difficult to remember all the normal variations for all ages, but by using growth charts with normal growth lines as shown, both the normal range and rate of growth can be seen easily.

People are often confused by the word 'percentile'. Looking at the chart on p. 49, the top line is called the 97th percentile. It shows the accepted upper limit of the normal range, and means that 97 out of 100 normal

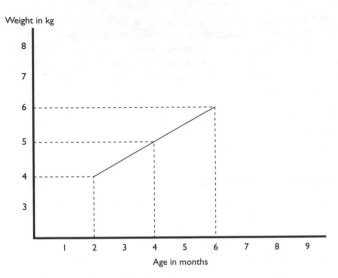

Figure 2.3 Normal rate of weight gain

children at that particular age will be lighter than this while three will be heavier. In the same way, the 3rd percentile is considered the lower limit of the normal range, and means that only three out of 100 normal children at that particular age will fall below this level, while 97 will be above it. Children below the 3rd percentile are 'at risk' and are termed 'underweight for age' (UFA).

In the same way, the 10th percentile means ten out of 100 normal children will weigh that or less and 90 will be heavier. It should be clear that the 50th percentile is the middle level; 50 out of 100 normal children will weigh less, and 50 more. It does not mean that 50 children will weigh exactly that, because there is a continuous range. You could see this, for example, in height. If you were to line up 100 seven-year-olds from the smallest to tallest, there would be very few of exactly the same size. The one in the centre would be on the 50th percentile, most would be of a similar height on either side, and a few at each end would be either very tall or very short.

The important thing is to remember that the normal range lies between these main lines (3rd and 97th percentile). Mothers should be told that this represents a path of health along which their children should climb steadily. If they see the weights plotted in this way regularly, they can

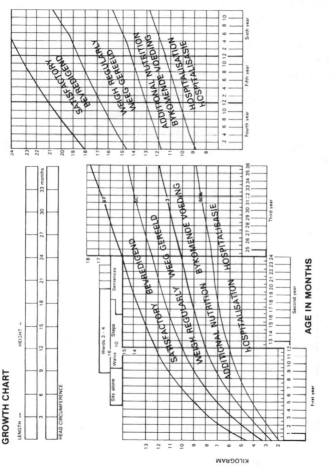

Figure 2.4 Example of a growth (Road to Health) card

be encouraged to take an interest and pride in their child's progress. If the baby's growth line either falls below this normal range or changes direction, one is alerted to look for the cause and take necessary action.

Uses and advantages of growth charts

Growth charts are used to check whether the child falls into the normal range for his or her age. Many children are found whose weights fall below the lower (3rd percentile) line. They do not necessarily look ill or obviously malnourished. They are just small for their ages, and if their weights were not plotted on growth charts, they would escape notice. These children are **underweight for age** (**UFA**) and represent the largest group of undernutrition. They are failing to thrive (see p. 56).

Recording growth repeatedly at intervals gives the most valuable information as to whether the rate of growth is satisfactory. The child's charted weight graph should run parallel to one of the normal growth lines given on the graph.

Parallel growth means good (normal) growth.

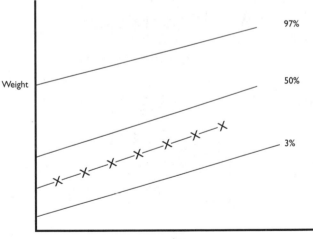

Figure 2.5 Normal parallel growth

If a child should have gained 1 kg over a certain period of time, but has, in fact, gained only 0,5 kg, this indicates a slowing of normal rate of growth, and is an early important sign of impending malnutrition.

Recording weight at regular intervals is of far greater value than any single recording, and shows what progress the child is making, that is, the pattern of growth.

Note: Plotting one position on the weight chart may be misleading, as it gives no indication of direction, whereas repeated recordings give both the direction and adequacy of the weight curve, which are more important in assessing progress.

Kwashiorkor may develop over a few weeks in a baby who was previously fat, but then suddenly deprived of protein and calories, for example breastfeeding stopped and only black tea / porridge given. The graph below (Figure 2.6) might be seen in such a case.

While most children with kwashiorkor register below the third percentile for weight, oedema fluid may falsely increase this weight.

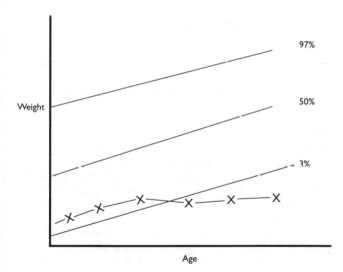

Figure 2.6 Flattening of normal growth pattern

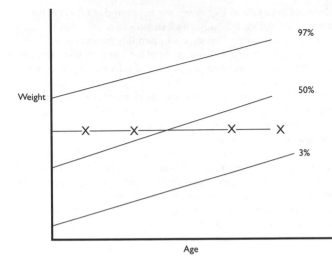

Figure 2.7 Abnormal pattern within normal range

A gain of 0,5 kg due to fluid retention will, however, show as obvious oedema. Because kwashiorkor can develop rapidly, the child may still be within 'normal' percentiles, but will have deviated from his or her previous growth curve (see Figure 2.7).

Infection and growth
In babies who are weighed regularly, and where growth charts are used, the relationship between infection and poor growth is noted.

Each time an infant has gastroenteritis or a severe respiratory infection, and particularly in the case of measles, there will be weight loss. Poorly nourished children tend to get more frequent infections, so one problem aggravates the other.

When recovery after an illness is satisfactory and complete, there is rapid regaining of the lost weight, that is, '**catch-up growth**', and the child continues on his or her previous normal growth line (see Figure 2.8).

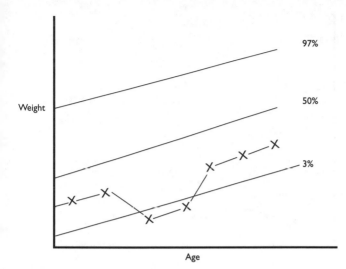

Figure 2.8 'Catch-up' growth

If 'catch-up growth' does not occur, for example after measles (see Figure 2.9), suspect some complication such as TB.

The growth chart indicates grounds for this suspicion, allowing for early diagnosis and treatment before the child develops serious lung disease, or even permanent brain damage from tuberculous meningitis.

Excessive growth

In infancy, particularly with artificial feeds and the early introduction of excessive amounts of cereal, a too rapid and marked weight gain can occur (see Figure 2.10). This is undesirable, as obesity develops which may persist into adult life, contributing to problems such as hypertension and cardiac disease. Obesity should be avoided in infancy and managed correctly.

Note: Comprehensive Road to Health charts are therefore used for all babies whether rich, poor, normal, overweight or underweight.

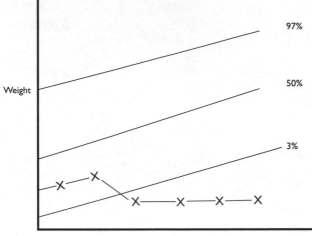

Figure 2.9 Failure of recovery

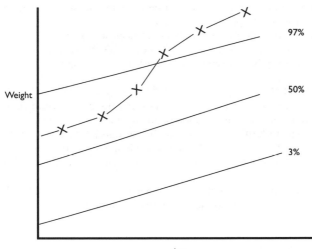

Figure 2.10 Excessive growth / obesity

The same comprehensive record must be used to document not only growth, but also immunisations, milestones of development, and other important information. This single form of card is a most useful and important document and the patient or parent must be encouraged to take it to all clinic and hospital visits.

In summary: the growth chart is used to:
- Determine and promote adequate growth.
- Detect children at risk.
- Introduce comprehensive health care to the family.

In a busy clinic, can time be found for all this? It must be found!

A growth chart detects which children need special attention and, through early intervention, can prevent serious malnutrition with the many associated severe illnesses. Children who fall below the normal range are considered at particular risk and are most likely suffering from malnutrition.

Weights are easier to measure than heights and show more rapid changes. Remember that weight, but not height, can be lost. Weight is therefore a more sensitive measure. Children should ideally be undressed when weighed. The scale should also be checked regularly.

Skull circumference is particularly important if some chronic brain abnormality (microcephaly) or abnormal growth of the head (macrocephaly) is suspected.

Apart from physical growth, the all-round development and progress for every child can be safeguarded. Malnourished children are inactive and learn less from their environment, while suffering more infections.

Classification of undernutrition
The use of charts enables all undernourished children to be classified by their position on the growth chart as well as the presence or absence of oedema.

Table 2.4 Wellcome Clinical Classification

Percentage of expected weight (Using 50th percentile = 100% expected weight)	No oedema	Oedema (Nutritional)
Between 60–80% of expected weight	Underweight for age (UFA)	Kwashiorkor
Less than 60% of expected weight	Marasmus	Marasmic kwashiorkor

This classification is traditional. The World Health Organization (WHO) is proposing a new classification based on symmetrical oedema, weight for height, and height for age. In this classification, standard deviation scores will divide children into moderate or severe malnutrition with additional sub-groups in the severe category of oedematous malnutrition, severe wasting or severe stunting. Another classification is that of Waterlow and is set out in Table 2.5

Table 2.5 Waterlow's qualitative classification of malnutrition based on height-for-age and weight-for-height

Category	Height-for-age	Weight-for-height
Normal	≥90% standard	≥80% standard
Stunted	<90% standard	≥80% standard
Wasted	≥90% standard	<80% standard
Wasted and stunted	<90% standard	<80% standard

Abnormal growth

Failure to thrive (FTT)

Definition

The term 'failure to thrive' describes a failure of expected normal growth and well-being. This usually occurs in young children (up to three to four years).

Clinical features

This problem is recognised by plotting weight on growth charts and:

- Noting those falling below the third percentile, or
- Noting those who have changed direction from a previously acceptable pattern of growth, that is, crossing percentiles, or
- Noting growth faltering, that is, when the growth curve is flat or dropping off for two consecutive months.

Features of undernutrition

The most important features are:

- Poor growth and development.
- Increased incidence of infection which is often recurrent or chronic.
- It always precedes frank kwashiorkor or marasmus.

'Failure to thrive' is not a diagnosis. It must be the start of a logical approach to find and manage the underlying cause. In addition to poor weight gain, many of these infants may also suffer emotional deprivation and lag behind in motor and social development.

While maternal and environment deprivation must be taken into account, it is best to use the term 'failure to thrive' to describe the group of chronically undernourished infants who suffer from a wide range of problems from simple starvation to chronic disease.

Physical growth depends on a number of factors. These are genetic, environmental, socio-economic, infective, emotional, and nutritional. The most important single factor is nutrition.

Aetiology

There are three groups of causes of failure to thrive:

- **Inadequate intake**:
  - Too little food given or
  - Too little food taken.
- **Increased loss** through vomiting or malabsorption.
- Poor utilisation of food secondary to an **underlying organic condition** (e.g. congenital heart disease), **chronic illness** (e.g. TB, renal disease, etc.) or, rarely, a **metabolic condition**.

HIV disease must be considered in all children who fail to thrive

Diagnosis

Approach the diagnosis of FTT in two stages:

1. A preliminary screening based on history, clinical examination, and measurements of weight, length, and head circumference. (Plot on growth chart.)
2. A trial of adequate feeding. This is best done in hospital. If done at home, close follow-up conditions are essential.

Preliminary screening

- Take a careful history with particular emphasis on events during pregnancy, the early neonatal period, social aspects, guardian-care feeding, vomiting, and stool pattern.
- Perform a thorough clinical examination to exclude serious underlying disease. Organic disease without signs or symptoms may remain undetected until the child fails to thrive. Certain congenital cardiac defects, such as a large ventricular septal defect, or renal abnormalities, may have escaped early diagnosis.

Urinary tract infection should be excluded by urine cultures, as it is often overlooked during other investigations.

Trial of feeding

Any plan of investigation must take into account that the majority of infants who present with FTT are suffering from undernutrition. Before all other diagnostic possibilities are considered, it is essential to establish that the infant is getting enough food and calories. A trial of feeding is best done under controlled hospital conditions, but this is often not possible and must then be closely supervised at home, with follow-up organised through nutrition clinics. It must take place over a period long enough to assess response, that is, two to three weeks. While this is happening, the performing of multiple tests must be avoided. Routine investigations such as FBC, CXR, Mantoux, urine cultures and stool for parasites can be done at this stage.

More detailed investigations are indicated if there is a poor response to a controlled trial of feeding.

Table 2.6

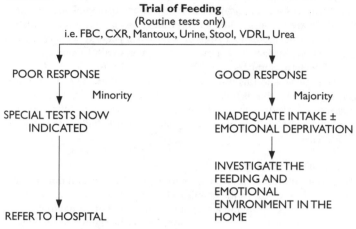

Management after trial of feeding

This is determined by the response to feeding. Adequate feeding requires a high energy intake, that is, 150–200 kcal/kg/day. This usually results in a satisfactory and often dramatic weight gain and indications of recovery. It usually takes several weeks for an infant to respond to an improved intake and positive emotional relationship. Attempts must be made to involve the mother in increasing contact with her improving infant. Close follow-up and supervision of the child are essential to ensure continued progress. If the child does not thrive despite getting enough food, referral for further investigation is indicated.

Maternal or environmental deprivation

This can lead to severe deprivation as shown by delayed physical, personality, motor, emotional, and intellectual development. Observation of mother and infant during a feed may be revealing. Feeding is the ideal time for physical and emotional interaction between mother and infant. Close contact, love, and security for the infant are essential for good feeding practice. Disturbed mothers may demonstrate total indifference, or even cold hostility, towards their infants during feeding. There will be a lack of eye contact and a minimum of physical, social, and emotional contact. The baby may also be relatively unresponsive. (Rumination should be considered in the case of any infant who vomits repeatedly with ease and satisfaction.)

The pattern of emotional deprivation is often one where the disadvantages and handicaps of one generation are passed on to the next. Solutions are not easy. Doctors and nurses faced with a malnourished infant must be careful not to direct feelings of anger and hostility towards the mother. 'Neglect' is a term which suggests wilful disregard for an infant's welfare. Some malnourished infants do have a history of neglect, or even abuse, and this must influence future plans. For the majority, however, the mother is unaware of her deficiencies in providing for her infant's real needs. She may have so many of her own difficulties and troubles, psychiatric or marital, that she herself is 'failing to thrive' as a mother.

Availability of services

An important part of prevention is to make health promotion services more easily available to the families who need them most, but use them least. This means bringing a programme of **preventive paediatrics** to such families. It involves regular home visits by figures acceptable to deprived communities, for example district nurses and health visitors, and setting up informal, friendly, and easily accessible neighbourhood clinics. It involves the training of nurses in tasks traditionally carried out by doctors, for example clinical and developmental assessments. The routine use of growth (percentile) charts at all clinics and hospitals is essential in order to detect those children who are failing to thrive.

Conclusion

Any serious attempt to break the cycle of ignorance, poverty, undernutrition, and deprivation must be both aggressive and positive. It must remove suspicion, overcome apathy, increase motivation, and demonstrate benefit. Socio-economic factors play the most important part in determining the quality of life for children in the community. This often makes management very difficult and relatively ineffective. Much can be achieved, however, if full use is made of available clinic services, nutrition clinics, health visitors, and educators.

Protein energy malnutrition (PEM)

The inadequate intake of protein and / or energy in the diet leads to this condition.

Classification

• **Underweight for age (UFA)**

In this category, the abnormality is that weight for age is below the lower limit of normal (third percentile). These children are generally not sick and often escape detection if their weight is not plotted on a percentile chart.

• **Marasmus**

The weight for age is below the 'Marasmic line' (60% of expected weight for age). These children are often ill and appear wasted.

• **Kwashiorkor**

Nutritional oedema is present. The child is usually below the third percentile but may occasionally fall within the normal range.

• **Marasmic kwashiorkor**

This is a combination of kwashiorkor, that is, oedema with weight for age below 60% of expected weight for age.

Underweight for age may be regarded as a mild form of PEM, while the other conditions should be seen as severe and life-threatening forms.

Causes

A diet low in energy and protein taken over a long period tends to cause marasmus. On the other hand, a diet containing rather more energy and less protein leads to kwashiorkor. In all cases, the problem is an **inadequate and unbalanced diet**.

Factors that lead to this include:

Social factors

• Unemployment of parents.
• Ineffective subsistence farming, made worse by drought and the high cost of seed and fertiliser.
• Sending children to stay with elderly unsupported relatives (usually grandmothers) in the rural areas.
• Administrative difficulties experienced by unsupported mothers and grandmothers in obtaining maintenance grants.
• Deliberate child abuse by parents or caretakers. Usually one child is singled out for abuse.

- Teenage single mothers who may be expelled from their parental homes without means of support.
- Failure of migrant breadwinners to send an adequate portion of their earnings back to their families at home.
- Socio-political: These factors affect all of the above.

Nutritional factors
- Breastfeeding not established post-delivery, or not maintained.
- Ignorance of caretakers about how best to spend their limited funds on foods with the best nutritional value (see Infant feeding, pp. 91–92).

Medical factors
A child who is chronically ill tends to eat poorly, which makes the problem of an already inadequate diet worse. It is particularly important to exclude TB in all cases of PEM. Measles, pneumonia or chronic gastroenteritis may also precipitate malnutrition.

Clinical features
Free radicle damage from free oxygen radicles can account for many of the features of kwashiorkor such as oedema, fatty liver, and excess mortality.

Kwashiorkor
- Characteristically irritable behaviour when disturbed, otherwise apathetic and withdrawn.
- Oedema.
- Thin de-pigmented hair.
- Dark peeling skin rash, especially over buttocks, perineum, legs, and lower abdomen.
- Angular stomatitis.
- Anaemia.
- Hepatomegaly.
- Muscular weakness and retarded motor development.
- Depressed cellular immunity leading to:
  - False negative tuberculin tests.
  - Increased incidence of TB, herpes, and monilia infections; HIV must also be excluded.
  - Gram-negative septicaemia.
  - Diarrhoea (aggravated by lactose intolerance and giardia infection).

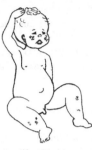
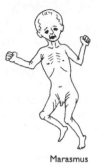

Kwashiorkor   Marasmus

Figure 2.11 Kwashiorkor and marasmus

Marasmus
- Evidence of marked wasting, including loose skin folds over the inner aspects of the thighs, buttocks, and anterior axillary folds.
- An alert anxious look in an old and wrinkled face.
- Oedema if marasmic kwashiorkor.

Management of PEM
In all cases, a full three-part assessment – social, nutritional, and medical – must be made so that all aspects of treatment can be planned.

Social
All possible helping agencies should be enlisted to assist. Lay (village) health workers, community health nurses (for home visits and follow-up), social workers (for grants and pensions), teachers, as well as ministers of religion are examples of people that might be asked to assist in specific cases.

Nutritional
- Promotion of breastfeeding.
- Education on the proper purchase and use of appropriate foods.
- Agricultural advice by qualified extension officers, and the promotion of domestic vegetable gardening.
- Provision of basic foodstuffs at subsidised prices, or free in specific cases. These foodstuffs should be what the mother herself would like to provide for the child if she could. Milk powder, beans, and coarse-ground mealie meal are examples.

Medical
- All cases must have a tuberculin test (may have a false negative result) and a haemoglobin level done.
- Children with kwashiorkor and marasmus should be admitted to hospital for rehabilitation if at all possible. The hospital treatment of these cases includes:
  o Prevent and manage hypothermia.
  o Antibiotics usually Co-trimoxizole or ampicillin / Gentamicin or cefotaxime or ceftriaxonne.
  o Blood glucose monitoring: Six-hourly for the first 48 hours.
  o Vitamin A 50 000 units orally before six months, 100 000 units six months–1 year, 200 000 units after 1 year given on admission.
  o KCl Solution, 6 mmol/kg/day until oedema resolved.
  o Milk feeds (e.g. Pelargon®) in smaller volume 80–100 ml/kg and given more frequently (three-hourly) by nasogastric tube, if necessary. If diarrhoea with lactose intolerance is a problem, start with soya milk feeds.
  o Treat for worms and giardia (Albenazole and Metronidazole).
  o Ward diet of solid foods when improving.
  o Folic acid 5 mg/kg/day for two weeks.
  o Multivitamin syrup 10 ml/day for three months.
  o Iron in the recovery phase (oedema resolved).

The duration of the stay in hospital is about 30 days. Children should not be discharged until they are above their admission weight and gaining steadily. On discharge from the hospital, the local clinic must be informed that the child is returning home so that staff can monitor progress and provide ongoing support. This is the most important phase in management, as it will determine whether or not the child recovers completely or relapses. Parental education is essential to prevent recurrence.

Some other important nutritional deficiencies

Scurvy (Vitamin C)

Ascorbic acid (vitamin C) deficiency is rare in southern Africa, as vitamin C is present in most fruits (especially citrus), tomatoes, and many green-leafed vegetables.

Clinical signs
- Swelling and tenderness of limbs due to bleeding into the muscle or under periosteum. This causes a pseudo-paralysis. Therefore, the child lies in a 'frog position' and is frightened of being moved (finds it painful).
- Redness, bleeding, and later ulceration of the gums in children whose teeth have erupted.
- Poor wound healing generally.

Treatment
- Prevention.
- Dietetic (fruit juices), multivitamin syrups, or ascorbic acid 250 mg orally six-hourly for three days followed by 10 ml multivitamin syrup daily for three months.

Rickets (Vitamin D)
- Failure in mineralisation of osteoid tissue at the end of growing bones. Only occurs in children who are actively growing (if not, growing deficiency causes osteomalacia).
- Most commonly results from a deficiency of vitamin D in the diet and a lack of sunlight.
- May also occur in liver and kidney disorders (rare).

Causes
- Inadequate vitamin D in diet (i.e. inadequate fortified milk, margarine, fish-liver oil).
- Too little exposure to sunlight (constantly indoors or 'wrapped').
- Preterm babies in their first year of life require greater amounts of vitamin D because of rapid growth (need 800 units/day while in hospital).

Clinical signs
- Rickety rosary at costo-chondral junction of the ribs.
- Craniotabes (softening of the cranial vault bones).
- Recession of chest on breathing (soft bones).
- Bossing of skull (forehead).
- Thickened wrists and knees.
- Harrison's sulcus (diaphragm pull).
- Bow-legs or knock-knees (only if weight-bearing).
- Hypotonic muscles and distended abdomen.
- Excessive sweating (mainly of head).

- Pneumonia is common and results from hypotonia with poor chest movement and recession of the soft thorax on inspiration (poor lung expansion).

Biochemistry

Alkaline phosphatase is increased; hypophosphataemia and calcium levels are variable and not always low.

Management

- Oral vitamin D 5 000 units a day for a month.
- Diet to include eggs, margarine / butter, and liver.
- Exposure to sunshine.
- Ensure 400 units vitamin D intake per day thereafter.

Prevention

- All preterm infants should receive 800 units vitamin D daily until discharge from hospital, then 400 units a day until six months of age.
- Adequate intake of milk.
- Exposure to sunlight.

Pellagra (Niacin / nicotinic acid [vitamin B. complex] deficiency)

This is a deficiency in nicotinic acid because of poor dietary intake of niacin or the amino acid tryptophan (from which nicotinic acid can be biosynthesised). It occurs mainly in areas where maize is the staple diet.

Clinical signs

- Desquamation dermatitis limited to areas of sun-exposed skin:
  o Arms and legs.
  o Face and forehead – butterfly distribution.
  o Neck (Casal's necklace).
    (Kwashiorkor, by contrast, has desquamation of buttocks and perineal areas, i.e. not sun-exposed.)
- Diarrhoea.
- Dementia (rare in children).
- Glossitis with fiery red tongue: Can lead to atrophy and insensitivity of tongue.
- Angular stomatitis.

Age
- Usually from ± five years.
- Children under three years usually have kwashiorkor as well.
- Found where basic diet is unfortified maize only.

Diagnosis
- On the clinical picture.
- Biochemical measurements.

Treatment
- Prevention: Niacin is a B-group vitamin found in liver, meat, fish, poultry, and green vegetables. Cereals are a poor source.
- Nicotinic acid 100 mg orally three times daily for a week.
- Improved balanced diet with sources of animal protein and / or beans, peas, lentils.

Xerophthalmia (Vitamin A)

Vitamin A deficiency in infants and younger children is often seen in association with PEM. Night blindness occurs in older children as well as adults.

Clinical signs
- The lacrimal glands stop functioning, which leads to dryness of the conjunctivae.
- Photophobia.
- Initial loss of transparency; later corneal ulcers develop.
- Keratomalacia: Softening and discolouration of the cornea.
- Night blindness.
- Follicular hyperkeratosis (dryness and scaliness of the skin).
- Lowered resistance to infection (measles, diarrhoea, etc.).
- Poor growth and dental development may occur.

Treatment
- Prevention: Vitamin A is a fat-soluble vitamin found in breast milk, cow's milk, butter, vegetables, and fruit (yellow – carotene).
- Vitamin A can be given by injection 200 000 units daily for two weeks.

Obesity

This is becoming a common nutritional disorder of childhood. The basic cause is that energy intake exceeds energy needs. Clinical criterion is a weight for height that is greater than 120%.

Hereditary factors

Overweight parents tend to have obese children. This relates more to family eating habits than to a genetic predisposition to obesity. There are also some syndromic and endocrine causes that need to be considered.

Environmental factors

- Sugar added to diet ('trained' to eat sweet things only).
- Early introduction of solids.
- 80% of bottle-fed infants gain weight faster than breast-fed infants. Human milk composition changes towards the end of a feed with the fat content becoming four times as much as at the beginning of the feed. This works as a signal for the baby to stop feeding, that is, an appetite controller (mother can't see what is in breast, unlike bottle, which then tends to be 'force-fed').
- Lack of exercise.

Problems

- Increase in respiratory tract infections.
- Delay in motor development.
- Knock-knees (when weight bearing).
- Emotional or even psychological disturbances.
- Obese adults: Problem of vascular disease (coronary artery / hypertension) and diabetes mellitus.

Management

Short stature with obesity is probably due to endocrine disease while a tall and overweight child is likely to have 'simple' obesity.

Management is difficult. Counselling, diets, increased exercise, and participation in sport must be part of a family approach to the problem, and all members must participate. Failure in trying to correct this complex problem is common.

Development

In order to assess whether a child is developing normally or not, it is necessary to have a basic knowledge of the main milestones of normal development. It is important to realise that for each milestone, there is a range of what can be considered normal. For example, it is normal for a child to begin walking at 11 months and equally normal to begin at 16 months. As there is a wide range of normal for each milestone, it is more useful to watch out for developmental warning signs which indicate the point beyond the uppermost limit of normal at which a milestone should have been reached.

If a child is found to be delayed in development, it is important to decide whether the child is abnormally slow in one particular aspect of development (for example, in speech it might be an isolated case of speech delay), or whether the child is delayed more or less equally in all aspects of development, as would occur in mental handicap or in multiple handicapping disorder.

Table 2.7

Developmental warning signs – Must be fully assessed	
Not smiling at mother	8 weeks
Poor head control	6 months
Unable to sit unsupported	9 months
Not crawling	12 months
Unable to stand with help	12 months
No spontaneous babbling	12 months
Unable to stand unaided	15 months
Not walking independently	18 months
Unable to understand simple commands	2 years
Not using two or three words	2,5 years

Disability

Prevention

The prevention of disability is a wide field, involving genetic counselling (to avoid Down syndrome, for example), reduction of maternal alcohol ingestion, the provision and acceptance of good antenatal and perinatal care, the achievement of high rates of immunisation, the control of tuberculosis, the ability to diagnose and treat meningitis, reduction in the incidence of gastroenteritis and particularly the avoidance of dehydration, and an improvement in road and household safety. In fact, the broad promotion of health in the community has a powerful impact on many causes of disability.

Ideally, every disability should be diagnosed as early as possible, so that corrective management and therapy can be started at a stage when the maximum benefit can be derived. Regular assessment of every child's developmental progress should be a function of primary health care services. This should take the form of simple developmental assessment at each clinic visit, and at least a screening test for hearing at nine months of age.

Common presenting complaints with disability:
- The child is delayed in sitting, crawling or walking, that is, delayed in motor development.
- The child is slow in all aspects of development (motor and social).
- The child is slow to talk (language development).
- The child experiences vision and hearing problems.
- The child repeatedly fails in the early grades at school.
- Combinations of the above.

In assessing a child with a problem in development, take a full paediatric history, paying particular attention to incidents that may have caused neurological damage such as:
- Problems with the mother in pregnancy:
  ○ Age of mother (remember that Down syndrome is more common in older mothers).
  ○ Did the mother experience any of the following problems during pregnancy: hypertension, diabetes, poor fetal growth, rubella, drugs or alcohol ingestion?
- Problems around the time of birth:
  ○ Was the delivery normal or was it by means such as breech, forceps, caesarean section, vacuum, etc.?
  ○ What was the condition of the baby at birth? Some useful questions to use in this area are:
    – What was the birth weight? If this is not known, ask simply whether the baby was very small.
    – Did the baby take a long time to begin breathing regularly, or did he or she need resuscitation?
    – Was the baby tube-fed for a period after birth? This may indicate neurological problems.

- Was the baby premature? The degree can be guessed from whether or not the baby was kept in an incubator, and from how long the baby spent in hospital after birth.
- Was the baby severely jaundiced? If so, did he or she have an exchange transfusion?
- Did the baby have fits in the newborn period?
- Were there any problems after the newborn period?
  Some significant past problems would include:
  ○ Severe diarrhoea with dehydration leading to a cerebral vein thrombosis.
  ○ Serious illness (needing hospital admission) such as pneumonia (during which the child may have had a hypoxic episode) or meningitis, resulting in CNS damage.
  ○ Head injury.

Family history
Developmental problems in other family members may indicate a genetic basis for the disability.

Developmental history
Most parents do not remember 'minor' milestones such as rolling over or holding the head clear of the bed. It is best to enquire about the major milestones, such as smiling, sitting unaided, standing, walking alone, and saying single intelligible words. Remember that there is never a fixed normal age for reaching a particular milestone; there is always a range of normality.

Upper limits of normality
Not smiling by eight weeks
Not sitting unaided by nine months
Not standing (supported) by 12 months
Not walking alone by 18 months
Only single words with meaning
at 36 months

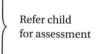

Refer child
for assessment

Delay in sitting or walking
The main causes of motor delay are:
- **Severe illness**: For example, a child recovering from kwashiorkor or measles may stop progressing in motor development for a period, or even go backwards; a child who was walking alone before measles or any other serious illness may not be able to do so afterwards.

- **Mental retardation**: It is usual that a child with mental disability will be more or less evenly delayed in all aspects of development.
- **Cerebral palsy**: This is a group of motor disorders caused by an insult to the brain around the time of birth or in early infancy. The five important types are:
  - Spastic (increased tone): 75%.
  - Athetoid (decreased or increased tone): 7,5%; often with abnormal movements (dyskinesia), especially of face and hands; severe cases have great difficulty with speech and feeding).
  - Ataxic: 5%.
  - Hypotonic (decreased tone): 5% often become spastic later.
  - Mixed: 7,5%.

  The disorder may affect one side (hemiplegia) or both sides of the body (quadriplegia) or mainly the legs (diplegia).
- **Rarer neuromuscular disorders**: These cause severe hypotonia (floppiness), for example spinal muscular atrophy.

Examination of the motor system

An approach to this is to carry it out in the following four stages:

1. With the child lying on his or her back:
   - Observe the child's position: In spastic cerebral palsy, the limbs tend to be extended, while in hypotonic (floppy) states, the limbs lie flat on the bed with the knees flexed.
   - Flex the knees and perform passive abduction with knees flexed and straight to test tone.

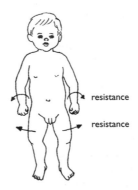

Figure 2.12 Test for spastic cerebral palsy

In spastic cerebral palsy, there is usually increased tone, especially on abducting the knees and supinating the forearms (see Figure 2.12).

In hypotonic states, tone is reduced and the limbs are floppy.

2. Pull-to-sit:
Start with the child lying on his or her back. Take the hands and gradually pull up to a sitting position. Observe:

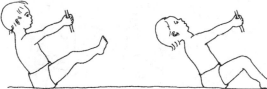
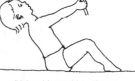

(a) normal before six months

(b) head lag and bent knees

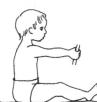
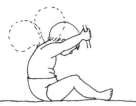

(c) straight back and knees normal after six months

(d) curved back and floppy head

Figure 2.13 Pull-to-sit

- The head: Does it loll back, stay in line with the body or come forward ahead of the body (as is normal after six months)?
- The curve of the back: Is it rounded like that of a newborn baby, or straight (as is normal after six months)? In spastic or hyptonic cerebral palsy, the back is abnormally rounded.
- Position of the hips and knees: The normal position after six months is seen in Figure 2.13c.
  In spastic cerebral palsy, the hips are at less than a right angle and the knees remain flexed. Head may be (a) normal position; (b) forward; or (c) hanging back in the young infant.
- Can the child sit unaided? This is normal after six to nine months.

3. Suspension:
Hold the child under the armpits and lift him or her clear of the floor or couch. Observe:

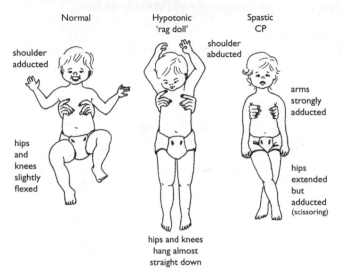

Figure 2.14 Vertical suspension

- Does he or she slip through your hands like a rag doll? This is typical of hypotonic states.
- The position of the legs: In spastic cerebral palsy, the legs and feet extend abnormally and tend to cross over each other. This is known as scissoring (see Figure 2.14). In hypotonic states, the legs hang down limply.

4. Walking:
If the child can walk, get him or her to walk up and down your consulting room or the corridor. Observe:

- Movements of the arms: Do they swing freely, as is normal, or does one arm not move? In hemiplegia, arm may be held at the side, or it comes up and is held in this position without swinging.
- The legs: In spastic cerebral palsy, the child may walk on the toes with a partially flexed hip and knee (see Figure 2.15). He or she may take very small steps, with the legs internally rotated.

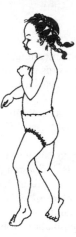

Figure 2.15 Spastic gait

Management of children with motor disorders

If the history and examination suggest a motor disorder, the child should be referred to hospital for diagnosis and treatment.

In the case of cerebral palsy, it is vital to begin physiotherapy as soon as possible. Such therapy can make a great difference to the child's final degree of handicap. The therapist usually sees the mother and child weekly for a prolonged period. Parents must be taught the techniques and exercises so that therapy can continue at home. In many remote areas, it is impossible for the pair to attend therapy regularly. In these cases, it is useful to admit the child together with the mother to hospital for a week or two several times a year. During these periods, the mother is taught the correct positioning and exercises for the child, which she then carries out when they return home. The therapist can also supply them with simple aids, such as positioning wedges and chairs made out of cardboard or other disposable material.

Children who are unable to walk eventually become too heavy for the parents to carry, and need a wheelchair. The collapsible and very light 'Buggy-Major' or similar model is particularly suitable, as it can be folded up for easy storage, fits into the boot of a car, and can be taken on a bus.

Delay in talking

Normal speech development

Ten months: Uses one word with meaning.
One year: Uses two to three words with meaning.
21 months: Joins two words; repeats things said; asks for food, drink, and toilet.
Two years: Uses 'I', 'me', and 'you'; talks incessantly.
Three years: Knows name and sex; uses three-word sentences.

Take a full history as above. Try to establish if there really is a significant delay, remembering that there is a wide range of normality. It is always abnormal to be using only single words at three years. It is important to ask about the speech development of siblings and parents, as benign delay in speech tends to run in families.

Carry out a full physical examination. This may reveal an associated handicap, such as cerebral palsy or visual impairment.

Remember that speech is learnt by imitation of sounds the child hears. If delay is present, consider the possible common causes:

- **Deafness or hearing loss**: It is essential to assess the hearing of any child with speech delay. Details of simple screening tests are given below. If your screening test suggests hearing loss, the child must be referred for formal audiometry at a centre (usually the ENT department of a specialist hospital), which has the necessary staff and equipment.
- **Mental retardation**: In such cases there will be evidence of major delay in most other aspects of development, such as motor and social.
- **Environmental deprivation**: A deprived or abused child who is not frequently exposed to the speech of adults and children will be delayed in speech development.
- **Isolated delay in speech development**: In this disorder, other aspects of the child's development, including hearing, are normal. It is an isolated disability, similar to dyslexia.

Management

This depends on the cause. With deafness or hearing loss, it is important to place the child in therapy as soon as the deafness has been detected. If this is delayed, the child may subsequently have great difficulty in learning to speak. Babies attend group parent sessions with speech therapists who teach parents how to stimulate their child. From three years onwards, the child may attend a special nursery school, and later a school for the deaf.

These schools are equipped with the appropriate apparatus and the staff are trained in teaching the deaf.

Note: The child with isolated speech delay needs intensive speech therapy.

The mentally retarded deaf child is largely managed as discussed in the section on mental retardation.

Screening tests for hearing loss
(See Ear, nose, throat, and mouth, p. 152.)

0–6 months
Observe if the young infant quietens at the sound of the mother's voice, or if he or she turns his or her eyes toward a sound.
6–12 months
The rattle test: See page 152 for details.
Older children
The easiest screening method is to get the child to repeat words that have been spoken (not whispered) into each ear at close range (10 cm). The Stycar screening tests are very useful when screening is done on a large scale. These require some simple equipment.

Note: Further advice and help about deaf or hard-of-hearing children can be obtained from the local branch of The National Council for the Deaf.

The child who is slow in all aspects of development
This situation usually involves mental retardation either alone, or in combination with other forms of handicap.

Causes
There are many, but the most common are:

Genetic	Down syndrome
Perinatal	Birth asphyxia
	Hypoglycaemia
	Kernicterus
Postnatal	Meningitis (including TB meningitis)
	Encephalopathy
	Head injury

Diagnosis

The developmental history and examination show general delay in all areas of development; that is, the child may be late in walking, talking, feeding him- or herself, and in acquiring social skills. In milder cases, it may be difficult to be sure whether the child is retarded or not.

Assessment of intellect

This may be difficult in the clinic or consulting room, unless the child is grossly impaired. In the child over three or four years, some idea may be obtained by asking about:

- Urinary and / or faecal continence by day and night.
- Ability to feed him- or herself.
- Ability to dress or help dressing him- or herself.

A further useful clinical test is the child's ability to copy shapes, which are first drawn out of sight of the child.

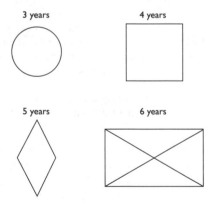

Figure 2.16 Copying skills

It should be noted that copying these shapes is not a test of intellect alone, but also of perceptual and other skills. It is nevertheless a useful screening test, which indicates when a child should be sent for more formal development assessment.

Management of the child with severe mental retardation
(IQ less than 50)

Stimulation and education
0–3 years
The child needs more active stimulation from the parents than the normal child. Parents often find groups consisting of other parents and children with similar problems very helpful. Toy libraries lend out suitable toys for a few weeks at a time, and provide support and advice to the parents on stimulation of the child.

4–6 years
The ideal environment is a 'normal' nursery school or créche. Here the child is stimulated by mixing with normal children.

7–18 years
Day training centre: Children attend daily and are taught everyday activities and social skills, such as how to eat at table, how to dress themselves, how to go to the toilet, and how to cross the road, etc. As they grow older, they are taught regular work habits in preparation for their adult placement in protected employment.

Institutionalisation
The most severe cases, who usually have multiple handicaps, are often best placed in a residential facility. Unfortunately there are long waiting lists, and this causes much hardship.

Financial assistance
When a parent stays out of work to care for a mentally handicapped child, the Department of Health and Welfare pays a single care grant. Two doctors must first certify the child under the Mental Health Act. The forms are then submitted to the local magistrate.

Additional handicaps
Attention must be given to these. They include seizures, behaviour disorders, incontinence, and constipation.

For further advice and help about mentally handicapped children, contact the local Mental Health Society in your area.

The child who repeatedly fails in the early grades of school

This is usually an educational rather than a medical problem, but certain obvious medical conditions must be excluded. About 3% of the population has an intellectual disability.

- **Mental retardation** (see above). In borderline cases, formal psychological testing may be needed for a definite answer.
- **Poor vision**. If a child has difficulty in seeing the blackboard, they need to be referred to the school eye clinic in your area for visual acuity testing, as they may well need glasses.
- **Poorly controlled epilepsy**. Frequent fits can disrupt a child's educational progress. With petit mal there may be many attacks per day, each one interfering with the flow of thought and learning. Refer to hospital for improved control and anti-epileptic medication.
- **Poorly controlled asthma**. Such children have many days away from school and concentrate poorly when they do attend. Ensure that medication is given regularly and, if possible, monitor the degree of control with regular peak flow measurements.
- **Deafness**.

If the above conditions can be ruled out, it is likely that the problem is either poor teaching, or that the child has a specific learning disorder such as dyslexia. In either case, the management is primarily educational, although occupational therapists are becoming more involved with the remediation of specific learning disabilities.

Genetic screening

All abnormal-looking children must be referred to a hospital for assessment. General counselling may be required, and investigations such as chromosome analysis and antenatal diagnosis in future pregnancies may be indicated.

Support groups

Intellectual disability

Mild (IQ 50–74)

Could manage mainstream education but would require additional special tuition which is often not available.

Moderate (IQ 35–50)
Special schooling for basic educational and life skills.

Severe (IQ 20–34)
Need constant supervision, eligible for care grants, and need placement in special care centres.

Ongoing support of families and their handicapped child is essential. Investigate and refer to known support groups (e.g. Down Syndrome Association) in your area. In many larger centres, a childcare information service is available, which provides information on what support is currently available, and how to contact different groups.

Chapter 3

Infant feeding

Nutritional education must start during the prenatal period and be continued at every clinic visit during childhood. This is particularly important in poor families where undernutrition is common. Good nutritional habits begin in infancy and are among the most effective preventive health care measures available.

Breastfeeding

Physiology

During pregnancy, the glandular tissue in the breast increases under the influence of the hormones prolactin, oestrogen, and progesterone.

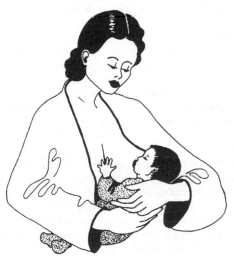

Figure 3.1 Breastfeeding

Colostrum

For the first few days after delivery, **colostrum** alone is secreted. Thereafter it is gradually replaced by mature milk. Colostrum contains a very high concentration of antibodies and immunologically active cells, such as macrophages and lymphocytes, and is an important means of providing the newborn infant with passive immunity. The small volume corresponds with infants' low fluid requirements in the first few days of life.

Mature milk

Mature milk consists of two main portions: the foremilk and the hindmilk. The **foremilk** is produced in the early part of a feed and is relatively dilute, containing less protein and fat than the creamy **hindmilk** which is produced later in the feed. Infants are able to regulate the dilution of the milk they drink by varying the proportions of foremilk and hindmilk. It is incorrect to think that the foremilk, which looks rather watery, is not suitable for feeding.

Prolactin

Between feeds, milk is secreted by glands in the breasts in preparation for the next feed. The quantity of milk produced depends on the amount of prolactin secreted. **Prolactin** is a pituitary hormone.

Prolactin secretion is increased by:
- **Sucking by the infant**: The more minutes per day of sucking, the more prolactin is produced; this is why it is important not to reduce sucking by giving 'complementary' bottle feeds.
- **Sleep**: Rest is important as it promotes prolactin secretion.
- **Lack of mental stress**: A worried, tense mother will secrete less prolactin than a comfortable and relaxed one.

Oxytocin

The release of milk that has already been secreted into the storage ducts of the breast is controlled by another pituitary hormone, **oxytocin**. Suckling is the most powerful stimulus to its secretion, but even the sight or sound of the infant may trigger oxytocin release. Oxytocin causes contraction of the myoepithelial cells (which resemble muscle fibres) surrounding the breast ducts, resulting in ejection of milk. Oxytocin does not stimulate the production of milk, but only its release.

Nipples

For satisfactory breastfeeding, it is essential that the infant takes the nipple and surrounding areola into its mouth. This requires correct latching. All mothers must be taught how to latch their infants.

The advantages of breastfeeding

- **Protection against infection**. As breast milk is sterile and contains both antibodies and immune cells, it provides protection against viral and bacterial intestinal infections, especially gastroenteritis. Breastfeeding also avoids the use of infected water and bottles.
- **Protection against allergy**. The fact that human milk protein is less 'foreign' than cow's milk protein accounts for the much lower incidence of allergic disorders in breastfed infants.
- **Protection against malnutrition**. Breast milk is always available when the infant needs it, even when the family cannot afford to buy other food. It cannot be diluted as is so often the case with artificial milk. Breastfeeding is cheap.
- Breastfeeding helps to **prevent malnutrition** even in the second year of life, as it will provide an important protein supplement to a staple carbohydrate food such as mealie-meal or samp.
- **Promotion of mother-infant bonding**. Breastfeeding brings a mother and infant very close together, especially in the early weeks when the process of bonding is most important.
- **Protection against breast cancer**. Women who have breastfed infants for a long time have a reduced incidence of breast cancer.
- **Uterine involution**. The oxytocin secreted during breastfeeding has a powerful effect on the uterus, causing it to contract, and undergo involution more rapidly.
- **Convenience**. Breast milk is always available, at the right strength and temperature, without needing preparation or sterilisation.
- **Birth spacing**. It is unlikely that a woman will fall pregnant if she is breastfeeding exclusively.
- Recent evidence suggests that **the intellectual development** is faster and better in infants that are breastfed.

Means of promoting breastfeeding

- **Early contact**. Newborn infants and their mothers are alert and seek each other within the first hour after a normal delivery. They should be allowed to have maximum contact in that period. Routine procedures that keep them apart (such as bathing) should be delayed for at least one hour. It has been shown that increased contact in this period leads to an increased length of breastfeeding, as well as better mother-infant relationships. Rooming-in post-delivery will promote bonding and help establish breastfeeding.

- **Avoid supplementary / complementary feeds**. During the first few days, the normal-term newborn infant has a low fluid requirement. This means that the rather small volumes of colostrum / milk that are produced are enough. Providing extra formula or water is usually not necessary, and only serves to reduce the amount of suckling on the mother's breast by the infant. This, in turn, reduces the production of milk. It also seems that it is easier for an infant to obtain milk by sucking on a teat than from the mother's breast. So, once an infant has experienced a teat, it may object to the breast. It is therefore best to keep teats and dummies away from breastfeeding infants. It is best to use a cup and spoon if extra feeds are needed.
- **Mother's nutrition**. For good lactation, it is important that the mother takes an adequate balanced diet and extra fluids.
- **Rest and relaxation**. It is very helpful if a mother can take a regular rest period during the day and get adequate sleep at night. Many mothers find it more restful and satisfying to have the infant sleep in bed with them. The dangers of 'overlying' have been greatly over-emphasised in the past.
- **Prolactin stimulators**. Certain medications have the effect of stimulating the secretion of prolactin. These may be used for a few days to re-stimulate a failing milk supply. Their use must always be accompanied by a good diet, extra fluids, and as much suckling on the breast by the infant as possible. These medications include meta-dopramide (Maxolon®). They must be prescribed by a doctor and should not be used for more than ten days. Frequent breastfeeding is the most effective way of stimulating milk production.

Common misconceptions about breastfeeding

- 'The working mother cannot breastfeed an infant'. If the infant is artificially fed by a caretaker during the working day, the mother can breastfeed during the evening, night, and early morning. Lactation is especially well maintained if the infant sleeps with the mother. Mothers can express at work to provide milk for the infant the next day.
- 'Small breasts cannot produce enough milk'. Much of the contour of a breast is made up of adipose tissue. Small breasts produce as much milk as larger ones.
- 'A short period of breastfeeding is not worth the trouble'. Many of the positive advantages of breastfeeding are of particular benefit to the very young infant during the first few weeks of life. These include the

anti-infective and anti-allergic effects. Therefore, even a period as short as two to three weeks can be of lasting benefit to the infant.

Common problems experienced with breastfeeding

- **Breast engorgement**. The breasts become generally enlarged, painful, and even oedematous on the second to fifth day after delivery. The milk flow is poor and mastitis is often incorrectly diagnosed. The correct management is to empty the breasts by manual expression or with a breast pump, and then to encourage the infant to suckle as much as possible.
- **Mastitis**. Not only is the breast swollen and painful, but the mother also feels unwell and may have a fever. Incomplete emptying of the breasts always makes infection more likely and should be avoided. Mastitis is not a reason to stop breastfeeding, and the infant can continue feeding from both breasts. Mild analgesia may be needed. Usually, treatment with flucloxicillin is adequate.
- **Breast abscess**. If an abscess has already formed, a fluctuant, painful mass will be felt in the breast. The patient needs hospital referral for antibiotics, incision, and drainage. Once the abscess has improved, feeding from that breast may be resumed.
- **Painful or cracked nipples**. This condition may be due to a variety of causes, including flat nipples, engorged breasts, and incorrect latching at the nipple. Do not advise stopping breastfeeding. The mother may need to express her milk for 24 to 48 hours to give her nipples a chance to recover. A protective cream such as lanolin cream, short spells of exposure to sunlight, and the treatment of candida infection (if present) all may help. The best protection for the nipple is a few drops of milk at the end of the feed.
- **Inadequate lactation**. The main causes of this are the use of additional formula feeds, missing out feeds, anxiety, fatigue, and contraceptive pills which contain oestrogen. Management includes ensuring adequate fluid intake and diet, rest and encouragement, frequent sucking, and possibly prolactin simulators.

Artificial feeding

Cup-feeding is currently preferred to bottle-feeding, as this reduces the risk of infection due to incorrectly cleaned bottles and teats.

Choice of milk

- From birth to six months, use a term formula such as NAN® 1, SMA® 1 or S 26® 1. The main advantage of term formulas is that they present fewer electrolytes to the immature kidney than formulas for older infants. Unlike breast milk, however, they do not provide protection against infection or allergy.
- From six months, use a full cream dried milk, for example Lactogen® 2, NAN® 2 or S 26® 2.
- From 12 months, either continue with full cream powdered milk, or use undiluted pasteurised cow's milk (if a refrigerator is available).

Other milks

- **Skim milk**. This is prepared from milk that has had most of the cream (fat) removed, which results in a powder that is high in protein and lactose. It should not be used as a milk feed in infants, but is very valuable as a high protein supplement to solid foods in older children. Skim milk powder sprinkled onto porridge makes a well-balanced energy and protein food. The high lactose content may lead to loose stools in infants with reduced lactose tolerance, such as those with kwashiorkor or chronic diarrhoea.
- **Soya-based formulas**, for example Isomil® 1 and 2. These milks all contain soya protein and are lactose-free. They have sucrose as their sugar. Soya-based formulas are prescribed for infants with intolerance to lactose. This is uncommon.
- **Hypoallergic formulas**, for example NAN® HA 1 and 2. These formulas are very expensive and should only be used in formula-fed infants with a strong family history of allergy or in infants with a proven allergy to milk formula.
- **Special milks** for chronic diarrhoea or malabsorption, for example Nutramigen®, Alfare®, Progestamil®, and AL 110®. These are used for specific conditions and should only be prescribed by a paediatrician or general practitioner.

Bottle hygiene

- Bottles should always be thoroughly washed with soap or detergent. A bottle brush is of great assistance. Teats should be washed and rubbed with salt and thoroughly rinsed. Then either boil the bottle and teat in a pot of water for ten minutes and allow to cool down before filling, or prepare a solution of Milton® or diluted Jik® and leave the bottles and teats submerged for ten minutes, or until the next feed. It is not necessary to rinse the bottle before filling it with milk. Teats perish very quickly when boiled, so rather use this method. To prepare the Jik® solution, place two litres of clean water in a suitable container, and add one tablespoon of unperfumed Jik®. This solution should be changed every day.

• If a fridge is available for storage, a whole day's feeds can be prepared together. Otherwise, make only one bottle at a time, as warm milk is a breeding ground for bacteria. Throw away any unfinished feed for the same reason.

Mixing feeds
Use clean, cooled, boiled water. Use one scoop (as provided by the manufacturer) for every 25 ml of water. Do not heap or pack the powder as this will produce an over-concentrated feed, and may lead to salt overload and hypernatraemia. The most dangerous error is to prepare a diluted feed, as the infant then receives insufficient energy and protein. This can result in growth slowing down, leading to kwashiorkor or marasmus.

Volume of feeds
After the first five days of life, 150 ml/kg/24 hours is usually adequate. The best guide to the volume of feeds is the infant's weight gain. Satisfactory weight gain is about 25 grams per day in the first four months, and 500 grams per month from five to 12 months.

The number of feeds per day
Infants under six months should receive not less than five feeds per day, while infants from six to 12 months should receive at least three feeds per day. Most infants will demand feed and decide for themselves when to feed.

Feeding of infants born to HIV positive women

The choice of breastfeeding or formula feeding in HIV positive women should be made before the infant is born. These mothers should be counselled to choose the most appropriate method for their infant. Formula feeding is only recommended in infants at low risk of death due to gastroenteritis and undernutrition. In addition, a mother should be advised to formula-feed only if formula is available and affordable, she has access to clean water, she is able to effectively wash mixing bowls, cups, teats and bottles, primary health care services are available, and formula feeding is acceptable in her community. Otherwise she should **exclusively** breastfeed for six months and then abruptly wean her infant. Continue with mixed breastfeeding only in very poor communities. Mixed breastfeedings (i.e. breastfeeding with other solids or liquids) carries the greatest risk of HIV transmission to the infant.

Feeding of solids to older infants and pre-school children

Food is needed in the body for three main purposes:

- The **energy requirements** of the body: This includes maintaining body temperature, the work done by muscles, and the carrying out of the many different chemical reactions involved in the body's metabolism. Carbohydrates (4 kcal or 16,8 kJ/g) and fats (9 kcal or 37,8 kJ/g) provide most of the body's energy. Proteins can provide energy if no other source is available.
- The **repair of tissues and cells** that normally 'wear out': That is, the hair, skin, blood cells, and cells of the small intestinal villi, etc. This process requires both energy and protein.
- The **growth** of the child and adolescent: This also requires both energy and protein.

If a child is not getting enough to eat, growth will slow down and, in severe cases, even stop completely. If the food intake is even further decreased, the processes of repair will stop. The skin will become thin, the number of red blood cells will decline, and the lining of the small intestine will become flattened. This stage is typically seen in kwashiorkor. The most severe case of all is when the energy supply fails. In this situation, the child's activity is reduced, the body temperature falls, and death is very close.

Food value of some common foods

- Energy-containing foods include carbohydrate-rich foods such as mealie-meal, samp, rice, sugar, and potatoes, and fat-containing foods such as margarine, cooking oil, and peanut butter.
- Protein-containing foods include beans and nuts, milk, skim milk powder, meat, fish, and eggs.
- Protective foods contain vitamins and minerals, but generally have very little in the way of protein or energy. Some examples include

green and yellow vegetables such as spinach, carrots, cabbage, squash, cauliflower, and pumpkin.

Important points about individual foodstuffs

- **Mealie-meal**: Under the large upper starch sac in the mealie seed is a small protein-rich germ bud. When the seeds are ground coarsely and the meal is left unsifted, a useful quantity of protein remains in the meal. The highly 'refined' and sifted meal usually sold in the shops has had almost all the germ bud removed. It therefore has a very low protein content. Samp is almost pure starch. It requires prolonged cooking. The fuel needed for cooking must be added to its cost.
- **Beans** are rich in both energy and protein, and are one of the most economical sources of protein.
- **Instant cereals**: These include Nestum®, Pronutro®, Cerelac®, etc. They are all scientifically prepared, pre-cooked foods and have excellent nutritional composition. Their major drawback is their high cost.

An outline of ideal feeding of pre-school children

Breast milk is the ideal from birth to six months. If necessary, formula feeds are used. For preterm infants and infants fed on formula milks which do not contain added vitamins, it is important to recommend 0,6 ml daily of a multivitamin preparation and 0,6 ml daily of an iron preparation. From six to nine months, start with a simple porridge. Later add vegetables one at a time, giving the infant time to get used to new tastes and textures. The quantity of solid food is gradually increased. The milk feeds continue as before but must be given after the solids. From nine months to four years, 600 ml of breast, artificial or fresh cow's milk per day is required. In addition, three or four good-sized solid food meals are given. The small stomach size of the young child makes it necessary to give feeds frequently. The most economical way to provide balanced meals at this age is to give a basic porridge such as mealie-meal, which should be mixed with small amounts of beans or skim milk powder which are rich in protein. Finally, add a small quantity of fat or oil. Some examples are:
mealie-meal + beans + cooking oil; or
samp + skim milk.
It is important to add vegetables to make these mixtures more palatable, and to provide vitamins, iron, and roughage.

The six golden rules of good nutrition for young children

1. Breastfeed exclusively until six months and then continue breastfeeding after starting solids until 18 months at least.
2. Start porridge at six months, not sooner.
3. Add protein and fat or oil to the porridge.
4. Give infants and toddlers four good-sized meals a day.
5. Give protective foods to children over six months.
6. A sick child needs to be fed as well as any other child.

Vitamin A

- Give Vitamin A routinely to all children from the age of six months to prevent severe illness (prophylaxis).
- Vitamin A capsules come in 50 000 IU, 100 000 IU, and 200 000 IU.
- Record the date on which vitamin A was given on the Road to Health Card.
- Vitamin A is not contraindicated if the child is on multivitamin treatment.
- **Note**: If the child has had a dose of vitamin A in the past month, do not give vitamin A.

Table 3.1 Routine vitamin A dosages

Age	Vitamin A dosage
Non breastfed infants (0–5 months)	A single dose of 50 000 IU at six weeks.
All infants 6–11 months	A single dose of 100 000 IU at six months.
All infants 12–60 months	A single dose of 200 000 IU at 12 months; then a dose of 200 000 IU every six months until 60 months.

The newborn

Examination of the newborn infant

All infants should be examined after birth to detect any clinical problems or to identify infants at high risk of developing problems. Give special attention to the following:

History
- Pregnancy duration, illness or complications.
- Duration of labour.
- Place and method of delivery.
- Complications during labour and delivery.
- Infant condition at birth; Apgar score if possible.
- Any resuscitation given.
- Feeding.
- Problems since delivery, for example jaundice, fits, respiratory distress.
- Any problems with previous infants.
- Blood groups, syphilis, and HIV status.

Clinical examination
- Routine observations: Weight, head circumference, and temperature.
- Assessment of gestational age if birth weight is low (under 2 500 g): Preterm infants can be differentiated from term infants by examining various external and neurological features (see Figure 4.2, p. 98).
- Plot weight and head circumference for gestational age on chart if birth weight is low (see Figure 4.1, p. 95).

General appearance
- Gross abnormalities.
- Colour: Normal, pale, plethoric, cyanosed, jaundiced.
- Rash or purpura.
- Oedema.

Head
- Shape: Moulding, caput, cephalhaematoma.
- Fontanelle: Open, closed, raised, depressed.
- Ears: Low set, misshapen.
- Eyes: Conjunctivitis, squint.
- Sight: Follows light or red object.
- Nose and upper lip: Cleft lip.
- Mouth: Cleft palate, teeth.

Neck
- Webbing of skin or thyroid enlargement.

Cardiovascular system
- Brachial and femoral pulses.
- Peripheral perfusion: Capillary filling time.
- Palpate precordium.
- Auscultate: Heart rate, murmur.

Respiratory system
- Respiratory rate and pattern.
- Any chest deformity or asymmetrical movement.
- Recession of chest.
- Inspiratory stridor.
- Expiratory grunting.
- Auscultation: Air entry, added sounds.

Gastrointestinal system
- Umbilicus: Infection, single artery hernia.
- Abdominal distension, redness or oedema of skin.
- Tenderness on palpation.
- Enlarged organs or masses.
- Auscultation for bowel sounds.
- Inguinal hernias.
- Anus: Site and patency.

Genito-urinary system
- Male: Site of urethral meatus, descent of testes.
- Female: Size of clitoris.

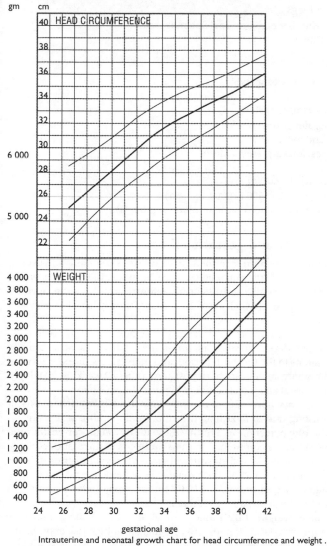

gestational age

Intrauterine and neonatal growth chart for head circumference and weight.

Adapted with permission from Lubchenco, L.O., Hansman, C & Boyd, E., *Paediatrics*, 37: 403, 1996.

Figure 4.1 Size for gestational age at birth

Arms and legs
- Arms: Number of digits, single palmar crease.
- Legs: Club foot.

Hips
- Dislocated or dislocatable.

Central nervous system
- Crying, alert, drowsy, asleep.
- Tone and movement.
- Reflexes: Sucking, grasp, Moro.

Placenta (If available)
- Weight (normally 500 to 600 g at term).
- Gross abnormalities (chorioamnionitis, infarcts).

Birth weight and gestational age

Normal infants are born at term (37 to 42 weeks of gestation) and usually weigh between 2 500 g and 4 000 g. Their birth weight falls between the 10th and 90th percentile and they are therefore referred to as **appropriate-for-gestational age (AGA)**. Term AGA infants usually have few perinatal problems.

It is not uncommon for infants to be born preterm (before 37 weeks or 259 days). These small, immature infants present with many complications in the newborn period, and therefore require special care. Less commonly, infants are born post-term (after 42 weeks or 294 days), when they are at an increased risk of hypoxia during labour.

Some infants have suffered intrauterine growth restriction or soft tissue wasting due to fetal undernutrition and are born with a weight below the 10th percentile as a result. These **underweight-for-gestational age (UGA)** infants commonly develop problems in the first days of life as a result of hypoxia and starvation before delivery. In contrast, other infants are overgrown with a birth weight above the 90th percentile. These **overweight-for-gestational age (OGA)** infants may suffer birth trauma and are often born to diabetic mothers.

Low birth weight (LBW) infants weigh less than 2 500 g. They may be born preterm, UGA or both. LBW infants are at high risk of problems during the newborn period.

Table 4.1 Assessment of gestational age: Helpful criteria in differentiating preterm from term infants

Preterm	Term
Ears flat and soft with poor recoil	Ears firm and well-folded along upper margin with good recoil
No breast tissue palpable and areola less than 5 mm in diameter	Breast nodule palpable and areola greater than 5 mm
Many vessels seen through skin of abdomen	Few or no vessels seen over the abdomen
Testes undescended or labia majora poorly formed	Testes descended or labia majora well formed
Skin crease absent or scanty over anterior third of sole	Many deep creases over most of the sole

The gestational age of an infant can be more accurately assessed by using both the external and neurological criteria of the Ballard scoring system (see Figure 4.2, p. 98).

High-risk infants

Neonatal asphyxia

Definition

Failure of an infant to breathe properly after delivery. The one minute Apgar score is less than 7, and the infant therefore needs active resuscitation.

Causes

- Fetal hypoxia.
- Airway obstructed with mucus or meconium.
- Preterm infant.
- Drugs given to the mother, for example pethidine.

Dangers

If adequate breathing is not started within a few minutes, the resultant hypoxia may cause heart failure, brain damage, and finally death.

Figure 4.2 Ballard scoring method

	0	1	2	3	4	5
Posture						
Square Window (wrist)	90°	60°	45°	30°	0°	
Arm Recoil	180°		100°–180°	90°–100°	<90°	
Popliteal Angle	180°	160°	130°	110°	90°	<90°
Scarf Sign						
Heel to Ear						

Score	Wks.
5	26
10	28
15	30
20	32
25	34
30	36
35	36
40	40
45	42
50	44

Skin	gelatinous red, transparent	smooth pink, visible veins	superficial peeling, and/or rash few veins	cracking pale area rare veins	parchment deep cracking no vessels	leathery cracked wrinkled
Lanugo	none	abundant	thinning	bald areas	mostly bald	
Plantar Creases	no crease	faint red marks	anterior transverse crease only	creases ant. 2/3	creases cover entire sole	
Breast	barely percept.	flat areola no bud	stippled areola 1–2 mm bud	raised areola 3–4 mm bud	full areola 5–10 mm bud	
Ear	pinna flat, stays folded	sl. curved pinna; soft with slow recoil	well-curv. pinna; soft but ready recoil	formed and firm with instant recoil	thick cartilage ear stiff	
Genitals ♂	scrotum empty no rugae		testes descending, few rugae	testes down good rugae	testes pendulous deep rugae	
Genitals ♀	prominent clitoris and labia minora		majora and minora equally prominent	majora large minora small	clitoris and minora completely covered	

Each separate criteria is given a score after examining that sign on the infant. These separate scores are then added together to give a total score. From the total score the estimated gestational age can be read off the table. Reprinted from *Journal of Pediatrics*, 95, p. 769, (1979), with permission from Elsevier.

Management

- Infants who do not breathe immediately after birth must be stimulated by drying with a towel.
- Keep the infant dry and warm.
- Clear the pharynx by gentle suction.
- If the infant still does not breathe, or has a slow heart rate, ventilate with a face mask and resuscitation bag, for example Laerdal or Ambu resuscitator. Only provide added oxygen if the infant is not pink within 30 seconds.
- Intubate the infant with an endotracheal tube if mask ventilation fails to provide good air entry (2,5 mm tube).
- Give cardiac massage if the heart rate remains below 60 beats per minute in spite of adequate ventilation.
- Narcan® 0,1 mg/kg, that is, 0,25 ml/kg (1 ml ampoules contain 0,4 mg/ml) IV, IM or *via* endotracheal tube for respiratory depression due to narcotics.
- Transfer immediately to hospital if normal breathing is not established within ten minutes.

Apgar scoring system

Asses the Apgar score at one minute after delivery and then every five minutes until normal. Each of the five clinical signs is scored 0, 1 or 2. The sum of the total gives the Apgar score (out of 10). Infants with a score of 3 or less are severely asphyxiated, while an Apgar score of 4-6 indicates moderate asphyxia. Normal infants score 7-10.

Table 4.2 Apgar scoring system

	2	1	0
Heart rate	100 or more	Less than 100	Absent
Respiration	Good	Irregular / gasps	Absent
Muscle tone	Active movement	Some tone	Limp
Stimulation	Good response	Some response	No response
Colour	Pink	Peripheral cyanosis	Central cyanosis

Meconium staining at birth

The mouth and pharynx of all meconium-stained infants should be thoroughly suctioned before delivery of the shoulders at birth (before the infant has a chance to breathe). Use an F12 catheter to remove as much meconium as possible. This may be a life-saving procedure, as severe lung damage may result if the infant starts breathing before the meconium is removed from the airways. Only suction meconium-stained infants again after delivery if they need resuscitation. Normal infants, who are not meconium stained and breathe spontaneously at birth, need not have their mouth and nose routinely suctioned.

Hypothermia

Definition

Skin temperature below 36 °C or axillary temperature below 36,5 °C. Usually measured over skin of trunk with a telethermometer, or in axilla with a digital or low-reading mercury thermometer. Normal skin temperature is 36–36,5 °C while normal axillary temperature is 36,5–37 °C.

Physiology of heat balance

Body temperature depends on the balance between heat production and heat loss. Heat is produced in the newborn infant by the metabolism of brown fat, other energy stores such as liver glycogen and subcutaneous white fat, and ingested milk. Newborn infants do not shiver. Heat is lost from the skin by conduction, convection, evaporation, and radiation. Subcutaneous white fat insulates against heat loss.

Causes

The following infants will rapidly become hypothermic if exposed to a cold environment:

- Wet infants after birth or after bathing.
- Preterm infants.
- Underweight for gestational age or wasted infants.
- Infected infants.
- Hypoglycaemic or hypoxic infants.

Clinical features

- The infant feels cold to the touch.
- Lethargy and poor feeding.
- A weak cry.
- Peripheral cyanosis, but centrally the body may be pink.

Dangers

- Cold infants rapidly develop hypoglycaemia, hypoxia, and generalised bleeding and may die.

Prevention

- Dry the infant well and keep warm at delivery or after a bath.
- Keep in a warm room, dress warmly or give kangaroo mother care if air temperature is low. Preterm infants may need incubator care.

Management

- Warm the infant in an incubator. If not available, warm the infant with kangaroo mother care and by heating the room with an electric or paraffin heater or open fire. Hot water bottles should not be used as an infant can easily be burned.
- Check the blood glucose concentration half-hourly, and treat hypoglycaemia which often develops while the infant is being warmed.
- When the infant is warm, dress well. If a transport incubator is not available, use kangaroo mother care or dress and wrap in silver swaddler or aluminium foil before transferring to hospital.

Hypoglycaemia

Definition

Blood glucose concentration below 2,0 mmol/l (or serum glucose below 2,5 mmol/l). Usually measured using reagent strips (e.g. Haemoglukotest®) with a glucose meter (e.g. Reflolux S®).

Causes

- Low energy stores, for example preterm, wasted, underweight-for-gestational age or starved infants.
- High energy demands, for example hypothermia, respiratory distress or infection.
- Abnormal liver function, for example hepatitis or hypoxia.
- Infant of diabetic mother.

Prevention

- Early milk feeds. There is no need for clear or dextrose feeds.
- Intravenous infusion with 10% dextrose if infant too preterm or sick for milk feeds.
- Keep infants warm.
- Use reagent strips to monitor infants at high risk of hypoglycaemia.

Clinical features

Often there are no abnormal clinical signs. The infant may be lethargic and hypotonic with a poor Moro reflex, poor feeding, apnoea, and cyanosis, or may be jittery and irritable with an exaggerated Moro reflex and convulsions.

Dangers

Hypoglycaemia may cause brain damage or death.

Management

- Mild hypoglycaemia with a blood glucose concentration of 1,5–2,0 mmol/l can usually be corrected by giving a milk feed. Repeat the blood glucose measurement in 30 minutes. Five ml sugar may be added to each 30 ml of milk.
- Severe hypoglycaemia with a blood glucose concentration of less than 1,5 mmol/l is a medical emergency and must be treated by starting an intravenous infusion with 10% dextrose if possible. Otherwise, give 2 ml/kg of 25% dextrose solution (50% dextrose half diluted with milk) orally followed by a milk feed with added sugar. Keep warm and give oxygen if cyanosed. Transfer to hospital as soon as possible.

Haemorrhagic disease of the newborn

Definition

Bleeding in the newborn infant caused by lack of vitamin K.

Physiology

The liver needs vitamin K to produce clotting factors in the blood. In older infants, most vitamin K is produced by bacteria in the large intestine. However, bacteria are not present in adequate numbers during the first week of life. Therefore, newborn infants have low concentrations of vitamin K and clotting factors.

Clinical features

- Bleeding usually presents between second and fifth day after delivery.
- More common in preterm, breastfed or sick infants.
- Blood in stool or vomitus.
- The infant may be very pale and shocked.

Management
- Prevent by giving 1 mg of Konakion® (vitamin K1) IM to all infants at birth. Oral Konakion® is not recommended. Those born at home are particularly at risk of not receiving vitamin K.
- If signs of haemorrhage are present, give 1 mg of Konakion®, oxygen, start IV infusion if possible, and transfer immediately to hospital.

Jaundice

Definition
Jaundice is a yellow colour of the skin and sclerae ('white' of eyes), caused by an elevated concentration of total serum bilirubin (TSB).

Physiology
Haemoglobin is converted to bilirubin which, in turn, is made water-soluble in the liver by conjugation, allowing its excretion into the bile. In the newborn infant, the liver is unable to deal with all the bilirubin and the TSB usually rises until about the fifth day and then falls. If the infant is not fed, the excreted bilirubin is reabsorbed from the small intestine back into the serum. Most normal infants develop mild jaundice during the first week of life (physiological jaundice), but the TSB usually does not exceed 275 mmol/l.

Causes
- An immature liver which is unable to conjugate and excrete bilirubin may result in marked jaundice in preterm infants.
- A delay in the onset of feeding which encourages the reabsorption of bilirubin from the intestine.
- Cephalhaematoma or extensive bruising leading to absorption of blood.
- The rapid destruction of red cells in Rh or ABO haemolytic disease.
- Infection, for example syphilis or septicaemia.

Important clinical features
- An infant with jaundice due to an immature liver appears generally well and is not jaundiced during the first 24 hours of life.
- Jaundice noticed during the first 24 hours is usually due to haemolytic disease.
- The presence of a rash, enlarged liver or spleen suggests syphilis while lethargy with poor feeding suggests septicaemia.
- A markedly raised TSB may not produce obvious jaundice in a dark-skinned infant.

Dangers

A serum bilirubin level over 350 mmol/l (20 mg%) may damage the brain and cause bilirubin encephalopathy (kernicterus). This presents with lethargy, poor feeding, opisthotonus, increased tone, convulsions, and may cause death. Survivors are usually mentally retarded with deafness and cerebral palsy.

Management

Infants with mild jaundice who appear generally healthy and feed well should be assessed daily until the jaundice starts to fade. Transfer the infant to hospital for further investigations and management if:

- Jaundice is noticed in the first 24 hours after birth.
- A previous infant had severe jaundice.
- Birth weight is under 2 000 g or the infant is preterm.
- Any sign of infection appears.
- The infant is lethargic or refusing feeds.
- Severe jaundice is present.
- TSB exceeds 275 mmol/l.

Most jaundiced infants needing treatment are given phototherapy. Some will need an exchange transfusion. Phototherapy must not be given to healthy infants with mild jaundice. Dangers of phototherapy include pyrexia (overheating), dehydration, and separation of mother and infant leading to failure of breastfeeding. A phototherapy chart is used to identify infants needing treatment.

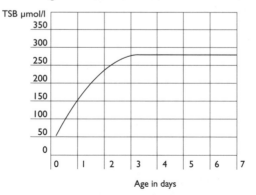

Source: Perinatal Education Programme: Perinatal Education Trust, Cape Town. Used with permission.

Figure 4.3 Phototherapy chart

Respiratory distress

Definition

A newborn infant with difficulty in breathing who has two or more of the following clinical features:

- Central cyanosis: A blue tongue in room air.
- Rapid respiration: More than 60 breaths per minute (tachypnoea).
- Grunting: A noise made during expiration.
- Recession (retractions): Indrawing of the ribs or sternum during inspiration.

Causes

Respiratory

- Hyaline membrane disease (immature lungs).
- Wet lung syndrome (delay in clearing lung fluid).
- Aspiration of meconium.
- Pneumonia.
- Pneumothorax.

Non-respiratory

- Hypothermia.
- Metabolic acidosis.
- Hypoglycaemia.
- Heart failure.
- Diaphragmatic hernia.

Dangers

Respiratory distress may result in hypoxia leading to heart failure, brain damage or death.

Management

- Keep infant warm.
- Give oxygen by head box or nasal catheter to keep tongue pink. If possible, measure the concentration of oxygen given and the infant's oxygen saturation. The latter should be kept at 86–92%.
- Provide energy with intravenous 10% dextrose or milk feeds.
- Check blood glucose concentration and treat hypoglycaemia.
- Give antibiotics if pneumonia suspected.
- Consider transfer to hospital immediately if the infant has hyaline membrane disease or needs more than 60% oxygen.

Examination of the gastric aspirate collected within 15 minutes of delivery is very useful in establishing the cause of respiratory distress. Pus cells and bacteria on microscopy suggest pneumonia caused by chorioamnioitis, while a negative shake test suggests hyaline membrane disease.

Convulsions in the newborn
Clinical features
May be generalised spasms, jerking of limbs, abnormal mouthing or eye movements, or even periods of apnoea without any abnormal movements.

Causes
- Perinatal hypoxia.
- Hypoglycaemia.
- Meningitis.
- Birth trauma.
- Congenital brain abnormalities.

Management
- Clear the airway and give oxygen if cyanosed.
- Check blood glucose concentration and treat hypoglycaemia if present.
- Give phenobarbitone 20 mg/kg IV or Valium® 0,5 mg/kg/dose rectally if fits are continuous or repeated.
- Transfer to hospital immediately.

Local bacterial infection

Umbilical cord (Omphalitis)
Clinical features
A wet or smelly cord often with periumbilical redness. May progress to cellulitis with skin oedema around the cord, or peritonitis and septicaemia, in which case abdominal distension, ileus, and vomiting will occur. Tetanus is an uncommon but important complication.

Prevention
Good cord care is essential for all infants. Clean cord three times a day with surgical spirits (or methylated spirits). Do not use powder or dressings.

Management

- If the cord is infected, clean at three-hourly intervals with liberal amounts of surgical spirits. Watch for periumbilical oedema or signs of septicaemia, peritonitis or tetanus.
- If present, start IM or IV penicillin and gentamicin and refer to hospital immediately.
- Prevent neonatal tetanus by immunising all pregnant women with tetanus toxoid.

Conjunctivitis

Clinical features

Discharge of pus from one or both eyes. Pus may dry and cake eyelashes. Conjunctiva becomes red and oedematous.

Causes

Gonococcus may cause severe conjunctivitis with oedema of the eyelids, with a profuse purulent discharge which usually begins during the first 48 hours of life. Other bacteria and Chlamydia usually cause a mild infection with sticky eyes, which often only presents 48 hours after birth.

Management

- Prophylactic chloromycetin or erythromycin ointment into eyes at birth is necessary in areas where gonococcal conjunctivitis is common.
- With mild infection, the eyes should be swabbed three times a day with saline, followed by chloromycetin ointment.
- With severe infection causing a profuse purulent discharge, use antibiotic drops or saline repeatedly to irrigate both eyes and to wash away pus. In addition, give IM cefotaxime 50 mg/kg and transfer to hospital immediately. Severe untreated gonococcal conjunctivitis may rapidly cause blindness.

Impetigo (Skin infection)

Clinical features

Impetigo presents with pustules of the skin. The infant usually appears generally well.

Causes

Usually caused by staphylococcal infection in newborn infants.

Management

Antbiotics are indicated only if there are features of generalised sepsis. Wash infant with chlorhexidine lotion and immediately rinse off with water. Repeat once daily until rash has cleared. Observe for signs of septicaemia. Staphylococcal pustules must not be confused with the common rash called erythema toxicum. This presents in the first week of life with red blotches that have small yellow centres. Erythema toxicum needs no treatment and clears within a week.

Generalised bacterial infection (Septicaemia)

Definition

Bacterial infection of the blood spreading to many organs.

Clinical features

- Preterm infants very susceptible.
- May start as a local infection, for example umbilical cord.
- Lethargy, hypotonia, poor feeding.
- Vomiting with abdominal distension.
- Apnoea or cyanosis.
- Hypoglycaemia.
- Hypothermia.
- Pallor.
- Continual bleeding from heel-prick site.

Management

- Keep infant warm.
- Check blood glucose concentration and treat hypoglycaemia.
- Aspirate stomach if distended.
- Head box or nasal catheter oxygen if cyanosed.
- Benzyl penicillin 50 000 units/kg 12-hourly and gentamicin 7,5 mg/kg/day given IV or IM daily.
- Transfer to hospital immediately for special care and antibiotics.

Congenital syphilis

Causes

The spirochaete *Treponema pallidum* may cross the placenta and infect the fetus. All pregnant women must be screened for syphilis (VDRL or RPR) and treated if necessary.

Clinical features
Mother
- VDRL or RPR positive.
- May have features of syphilis with rash, mouth ulcers, fever, enlarged liver and spleen.
- Treat with 2,4 million units benzathine penicillin IM weekly for three weeks. If possible, last dose must be given more than a month before delivery.

Infant
- Often low birth weight.
- Lethargic and feeds poorly.
- Peeling skin on hands and feet, often with blisters.
- Pale and jaundiced.
- Purpura common.
- Enlarged liver and spleen with distended abdomen.
- Pseudoparesis of one or more limbs.
- Metaphysitis on X-ray of long bones.
- May have no clinical signs at all.

Placenta
- Usually heavy and pale.

Treatment
- If clinical features of syphilis are present, give procaine penicillin 50 000 units/kg IM daily for ten days.
- If no clinical features are present, give benzathine penicillin 50 000 units/kg IM once only.

Rubella (Congenital rubella syndrome)
If a woman is infected with rubella during pregnancy, the virus may cross the placenta and infect her fetus, causing the congenital rubella syndrome. Fetal infection in the first trimester is usually severe and may cause congenital heart abnormalities, deafness, and blindness.

Clinical features
With mild fetal infection, the newborn infant may appear normal. However, with severe infection, the infant is growth-restricted, pale and jaundiced with hepatosplenomegaly, bleeding tendency, and rash. The infant may also have microcephaly, cataracts, patent ductus arteriosus, and nerve deafness. Most severely infected infants die, while survivors

are mentally retarded. Rubella virus can be cultured from the throat and urine. The risk of the fetus developing the rubella syndrome is greatest in the first trimester. Later infection may cause deafness only.

Management
The best treatment is prevention by immunising all children. Anyone suffering from rubella should be kept away from pregnant women.

Common minor problems

Cephalhaematoma
Definition
A collection of blood over the skull between the periosteum and the parietal bone. Typically limited by the periosteum at outer margins of bone. Caused by birth trauma. No treatment is needed for a cephalhaematoma. Do not aspirate.

Clinical features
- Common.
- Usually unilateral.
- Fluctuant.
- May cause jaundice due to the absorption of the blood.
- Infant appears generally healthy.
- May take months to disappear completely.

Not to be confused with:
- Caput over the 'presenting part', which is boggy, non-fluctuant, and clears within 48 hours. It may be marked after vacuum extraction.
- Subaponeurotic bleed which is massive bleeding under the scalp resulting in a pale, shocked infant with an enlarging, generally boggy head. Resuscitate, start IV fluid, and transfer to hospital immediately for blood transfusion.

Enlarged breasts
- Newborn infants, male and female, often have enlarged breasts due to the high oestrogen concentration in the fetus. The breasts must not be squeezed, as this introduces infection. They return to normal within a few weeks.
- If the breast is red and oedematous, an abcess has formed. Refer to hospital immediately for antibiotics and drainage.

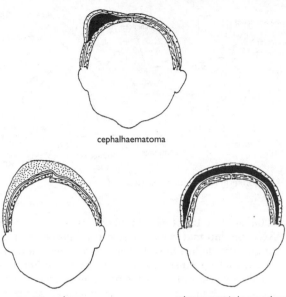

cephalhaematoma

caput succedaneum   subaponeurotic haemorrhage

Figure 4.4 Caput, cephalhaematoma, and subaponeurotic bleed

Mucoid or bloody vaginal discharge
Common in the first ten days of life and is also due to high hormone concentrations. Requires no treatment. Disappears spontaneously. Reassure mother.

Tongue-tie
The neonate often has a relatively short lingual frenulum (membrane under the tongue) which elongates in the course of one to two years. It is impossible for the child to stick his or her tongue out beyond the lower incisor teeth. Problematic tongue-tie is very rare and should not be diagnosed under one year.

Common congenital abnormalities

Congenital dislocation of the hip
Some infants, especially girls delivered in a breech position, have a

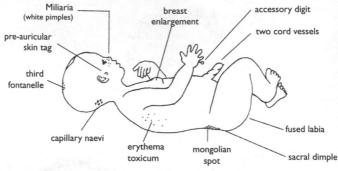

Figure 4.5 Common minor abnormalities

dislocated hip at birth. If not recognised and treated by splinting soon after delivery, the hip may remain dislocated, causing great difficulty with walking in later life. The hips of all newborn infants should therefore be examined to exclude a dislocated or dislocatable hip. This is done by flexing the hips and knees while the infant is in the supine position. With the examiner's thumb in front of the femur and the fingers behind, the femoral head is gently rocked forwards and backwards (Barlow's test). If the femoral head is felt to move forward into the acetabulum, the hip is dislocated and the infant must be referred urgently to hospital for further evaluation. If the hip can be pushed backwards out of the acetabulum, it is dislocatable. These infants should also be referred if the hip is still dislocatable two weeks after delivery.

Cleft lip and palate
Occasionally infants are born with a cleft lip, palate, or both. These infants may have severe feeding problems, as they are sometimes unable to suck well and have to be fed by cup, spoon, or bottle with a large hole cut or burned in the teat. They often breastfeed easily. They should be referred to hospital for assessment. The cleft lip and palate are surgically corrected within months of delivery. As they grow older, many children with a cleft palate have speech problems and recurrent ear infections.

Club foot
Either one or both feet are abnormal. The foot is twisted inward, points down, and is shortened. It cannot be pulled into a normal position. In contrast, many infants have feet that look abnormal due to the position

they have adopted before birth. However, these feet can be twisted easily into a normal position and need no treatment. All true clubbed feet must be referred to hospital as soon as possible after delivery. Treatment initially is by splinting in plaster of Paris. Later it may be necessary to operate. Delayed treatment results in permanently deformed feet.

Surgical emergencies in the newborn

Infants born with congenital abnormalities must be transferred to hospital immediately. Congenital abnormalities are often multiple. If you notice a minor abnormality, always examine the infant carefully for a major abnormality. The following major abnormalities can be recognised at birth:

Oesophageal atresia

Pregnancy is often complicated by polyhydramnios. At delivery, these infants appear to have a lot of saliva, as they are unable to swallow. They soon develop respiratory distress due to the reflux of gastric contents *via* a fistula into the lungs as well as aspiration of feeds. The diagnosis is confirmed if a nasogastric tube cannot be passed into the stomach. These infants must be nursed with their head elevated to prevent gastric reflux, must not be fed by mouth, and should receive oxygen if they become cyanosed. Transfer to hospital immediately.

Ano-rectal malformation

These infants have no anus and rapidly develop abdominal distension after delivery. They may pass meconium through a fistula into the vagina in girls or bladder in boys. Mild cases require a minor operation to open the anus, but severe cases need an ileostomy and later major surgery. Refer to hospital as soon as possible.

Meningomyelocele (Neural tube defect)

These infants have a major abnormality of the spine, with an area of spinal cord exposed on the surface of the skin over the back. The infant may also have hydrocephalus and usually has paralysed legs, no anal tone, and dribbles urine. The **meningomyelocele** should be covered with sterile gauze or a plastic packet to prevent infection during transport. Urgent transfer to hospital for assessment is needed. The outcome depends on the severity of the malformation. **Anencephaly** is a very severe form of neural tube defect. The top of the skull and part of the brain are absent and all infants with this defect die soon after delivery. The risk of recurrence of all neural tube defects in future pregnancies can be reduced by taking oral folate before and after conception.

Omphalocoele and gastroschisis

These conditions are both defects in the anterior abdominal wall, allowing bowel and often the liver to herniate out of the abdominal cavity. An **omphalocoele** is central and gives rise to the umbilical cord. The abdominal contents are covered by a thin walled sac which may perforate. In contrast, a **gastroschisis** is situated to the side of the umbilical cord and the abdominal contents are not covered by a membrane. An omphalocoele is often associated with other congenital abnormalities. In both conditions, the protruding bowel should be covered with sterile gauze or a plastic packet. Do not try to replace the bowel into the abdominal cavity. Refer the infant to hospital urgently for surgical correction.

Transferring newborn infants

Infants must be fully resuscitated before they are moved. Before transferring a small or sick infant to hospital, it is essential to contact the receiving doctor and discuss the problem. If possible, the receiving hospital should then send staff to collect the infant. While being transported, the infant should be kept in the optimal condition. The most common complications on the way to hospital are hypothermia, hypoglycaemia, and hypoxia. The infant should be warmed up to 36 °C before being moved, and then kept warm in a transport incubator or by kangaroo mother care. If neither is available, dress the infant in warm clothes and then wrap in silver swaddler or aluminium foil. Hypoglycaemia is best prevented by starting a 10% dextrose infusion. If this is not possible, a small milk feed can be given *via* a nasogastric tube. Cyanosed infants must be given enough oxygen to keep the tongue pink. If the infant stops breathing, face mask ventilation must be given. Monitor the infant's temperature, colour, breathing, and blood glucose concentration during transport. If possible, the mother should accompany the infant. If this is not possible, consent for any surgery required should be obtained before transferring the patient. It is essential that a referral letter giving all relevant details be sent with the infant.

Chapter 5

Cardiovascular system

Heart disease in children will present at primary care level in one of three ways. These are as:
- A heart murmur found on examination.
- Heart failure.
- Congenital heart disease.

Cardiac murmurs

A heart murmur is the noise caused by blood flowing through abnormal valves or defects in heart walls or a patent ductus arteriosis (PDA). For example, a narrowed valve (stenosis) will lead to a murmur being generated by the blood flowing through it. A defect (hole) in the wall between the ventricles such as occurs in a congenital lesion such as ventriculoseptal defect (VSD), will similarly cause a murmur as blood streams from one side of the defect to the other during cardiac contraction. In some children, soft, innocent murmurs occur in a completely normal heart.

Significance of a heart murmur

A murmur may be 'innocent', in other words, it occurs in a normal heart and hence requires no further attention. On the other hand, a murmur may occur because the heart is abnormal in some way. There may sometimes be other clinical clues which suggest that the murmur is significant. For example, the baby may have repeated chest infections, or may have very poor growth due to a congenital heart defect. Because there is no reliable way of making the distinction between an innocent and a significant murmur at primary care level, it is sound policy to refer children with newly discovered murmurs to hospital for evaluation. This will involve chest X-rays, ECGs, and expert opinion.

Cardiac failure

Cardiac failure occurs when the output of the heart is inadequate for the needs of the body. In adults, it is typically associated with shortness of breath, oedema of the legs, and (in severe cases) with pulmonary oedema causing severe respiratory distress. In older children, the picture is very similar, but in babies and young children it is the respiratory symptoms that dominate the clinical picture. A small baby developing cardiac failure will become increasingly tachypneic, and will have difficulty in feeding as

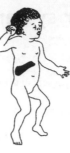

Signs:
Rapid respiratory rate
Enlarged heart
Thrill or murmur
Enlarged liver

Symptoms:
Breathlessness,
especially on
feeding or crying
Sweating

Figure 5.1 Cardiac failure

a result. As the condition worsens, the baby will develop an enlarged liver, become oedematous, and finally develop cyanosis.

Manifestations of cardiac failure in infants
Causes
- Severe congenital heart abnormalities, such as a large ventriculoseptal defect.
- Patent ductus arteriosis, especially in preterm infants.
- Viral infection of the myocardium (myocarditis).

Clinical features of cardiac failure in infants
- Feeding poorly.
- Tachypnoea with recession.
- Tachycardia.
- A murmur may be present.
- Cyanosis.
- Sweating (especially of the head).
- Weight gain (fluid retention).
- Enlarged liver.
- Oedema of the lower legs and / or face (late sign).

Manifestations of cardiac failure in older children
Causes
- Acute rheumatic fever.
- Established rheumatic heart disease.
- Acute glomerulonephritis: Failure occurs as a result of fluid overload and hypertension.

- Viral myocarditis in which the heart muscle is weakened by infection.
- Congenital heart disease.
- Other.

Clinical features
- Fatigue.
- Shortness of breath, particularly on effort.
- Repeated chest infections.
- Poor growth or developmental delay.
- Raised jugular venous pressure.
- Tachypnoea.
- Soft, tender, enlarged liver.
- Oedema (late sign).
- Gallop rhythm.

Treatment of cardiac failure (at all ages)
- Limit activities that cause stress.
- Oxygen.
- Nurse with head of the bed raised.
- Urgent referral to hospital for diuretic, digoxin, and other treatment.
- Reassure child and parents.

Congenital heart disease
Babies may be born with one or more of a large number of different anatomical abnormalities of the heart. There are four main ways that congenital heart disease will present:

1. As the incidental finding of a murmur in an otherwise well baby or child: an example would be a small ventriculoseptal defect.
2. As a baby or child with poor growth and repeated chest infections: these patients will usually have a murmur as well; examples would be a large ventriculoseptal defect or patent ductus arteriosis.
3. As a baby with cyanosis from soon after birth: this cyanosis is not relieved by oxygen therapy; an example would be the tetralogy of Fallot.
4. As cardiac failure, usually in infancy: an example would be coarctation of the aorta.

Management is as for any associated condition, such as cyanosis or cardiac failure, followed by referral for investigation.

Cyanosis

Cyanosis is due to unoxygenated haemoglobin in the blood. Haemoglobin without oxygen attached to it has a 'blue' colour. It may be peripheral or central.

Peripheral cyanosis

- This is noted in the extremities when the circulation is poor, for example as a result of shock or cold.
- When the blood circulates slowly, more oxygen than normal is removed by the tissues, and this results in peripheral cyanosis.
- Areas commonly affected are the hands, feet, ears, cheeks, and lips.
- It does not always indicate disease, as it may occur in cold weather.
- Always look carefully for central cyanosis.

Central cyanosis

This is best seen in the tongue, as the colour of the mucous membranes of the mouth and eyes may be unreliable. The oxygen saturation is abnormally low (under 90%).

Causes

- Cardiac failure (severe), from any cause.
- Cyanotic congenital heart disease, in which case the child may not be acutely distressed.
- Right to left shunt or common mixing disorder.
- Severe lung disease, such as pneumonia or bronchiolitis, in which case the child will be severely distressed.

The hands and feet are cold in peripheral cyanosis and usually warm in central cyanosis.

Management

Peripheral cyanosis

- Warm the patient.
- Reassure parents.
- Supportive measures; IV fluids for shock, etc.

Central cyanosis

- Refer urgently.
- Give oxygen even though this may not improve cyanosis if it is due to cyanotic heart disease.

Note: Central cyanosis is an indication for urgent referral.

Heart murmurs

Heart murmurs may be:
- Innocent or functional:
  - These are common, but a murmur can only be classified as innocent after expert medical examination.
- Organic:
  - Due to underlying heart disease.

Types of murmurs

- **Systolic:** Grade 1–6, classified by loudness and presence or absence of a thrill.
- **Diastolic:** Grade 1–4, classified by loudness and presence or absence of a thrill.

A murmur which is felt with the flat of the hand on the chest wall is called a thrill. This may be a systolic or diastolic thrill. If a systolic thrill is felt, the murmur is graded as 4/6 or greater. If a diastolic thrill is felt, the murmur is graded as 3/4 or greater.

Areas in which to listen for murmurs originating from the different valves or common congenital heart defects:

Mitral valve	Apex of heart and radiating to axilla
Pulmonary valve	2 left intercostal space (LICS) sternal border
Aortic valve	2 right intercostal space (RICS) sternal border
Tricuspid valve	4 RICS sternal border
PDA	2 LICS sternal border and radiating up to left clavicle
VSD	4 LICS sternal border

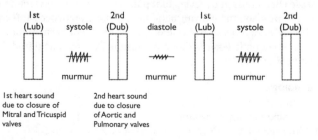

Figure 5.2 Timing on auscultation of sounds and murmurs

Assessment and management of a child in whom a heart murmur is found

History

Check especially for:
- A history of feeding problems.
- Failure to thrive.
- Developmental progress.
- Recurrent chest infections.

Examination (apart from the cardiac murmur)
- Check for tachypnoea or tachycardia.
- Cyanosis or finger clubbing.
- Jugular venous pressure.
- Hepatomegaly.
- Femoral pulses.
- Signs of chest infection.
- Haemoglobin level.

Chest X-ray

May show cardiomegaly.

ECG

Refer all children with cardiac murmurs for full assessment. If cardiac failure is present as well, refer urgently.

Rheumatic fever

Definition

A disease characterised by fever, joint pains, and heart involvement, due to an immune reaction following beta-haemolytic streptococcal infection. This disease is significant because of the possibility of permanent heart damage. Rheumatic fever is the most common cause of acquired heart disease in South Africa.

Epidemiology

More common in:
- Lower socio-economic groups.
- Children aged five to 15 years.
- Overcrowded houses.
- Delay in treating throat infections.

Cause

A poorly understood hypersensitivity reaction to the beta-haemolytic streptococcus. The condition develops some three weeks after the onset of a beta-haemolytic streptococcal throat infection.

Prevention

- Overcrowded housing conditions promotes the spread of beta-haemolytic streptococcal infections. The development of appropriate mass housing programmes is critical in the prevention of acute rheumatic fever.
- The early diagnosis and adequate antibiotic treatment of streptococcal throat infections in the community will lead to a reduction in the number of cases of acute rheumatic fever. This implies the development of an easily accessible health service capable of providing this care.
- Penicillin prophylaxis in children who have already suffered one attack is essential to avoid the recurrences which are a major problem with this condition.

Clinical features

The clinical picture includes some of the following:
- Pharyngitis or tonsillitis three weeks previously.
- Low-grade fever.
- Pain in large joints of the arms and legs lasting about 24 hours, then moving to other joints (arthralgia); this may develop into full-blown arthritis with swelling and warmth.
- Facial pallor.
- Tachycardia at rest and during sleep.
- Cardiac murmur.
- Subcutaneous nodules on extensor surfaces of joints (seen when joints are flexed) or over pressure points, such as the scapulae or occiput.
- Erythema marginatum (a very uncommon rash).

Diagnosis of acute rheumatic fever

Modified Duckett-Jones criteria are helpful in the diagnosis of acute rheumatic fever.

- Major criteria:
  - Carditis (murmur).

- o Migrating polyarthritis, which usually affects the large joints, for
  example knees, ankles, elbows (objective).
- o Subcutaneous nodules especially over bony prominences.
- o Erythema marginatum.
- o Chorea (abnormal, jerky movements).
- Minor criteria:
  - o History of previous acute rheumatic fever or signs of established
    rheumatic heart disease.
  - o Arthralgia: Joint pain, but no warmth or swelling (subjective).
  - o Raised erythrocyte sedimentation rate (ESR).
  - o Leucocytosis.
  - o Prolonged PR interval on ECG.
  - o Fever.
  - o Raised C-reactive protein

The diagnosis depends on a minimum of:
- Two major signs + evidence of recent streptococcal infection (such as
  raised serum ASO titre or positive culture on throat swab)
  or
- One major + two minor signs + evidence of recent streptococcal
  infection.

In view of the long-term implications of prolonged penicillin prophylaxis,
the diagnosis should not be made lightly.

Investigations at hospital level would include a throat swab, ESR, ASO
titre, chest X-ray, and ECG. Bacterial endocarditis must be excluded.

Course of illness
This is prolonged (± six weeks). The fever gradually subsides, as do the
joint pains and the cardiac murmurs. Residual joint damage is rare. Long-
term sequelae in the heart such as mitral incompetence are common, and
may lead to mitral stenosis years later from severe damage to the mitral
valve, especially with repeated acute attacks of rheumatic fever.

Management
Any patient suspected of having rheumatic fever should be referred to
hospital for a definite diagnosis. Initial management should be in hospital
and includes:
- Bed rest: Be creative and provide age-appropriate activities which can
  be done while resting to keep the child occupied; reassure child, as
  bed rest can provoke anxiety.
- Penicillin V 250 mg six-hourly for ten days to eradicate streptococcal
  infection.

- Aspirin (Disprin®): For fever and joint pains.
- Corticosteroids may help if there is active involvement of the heart, that is, carditis.
- Digoxin and Lasix® if cardiac failure occurs.
- Monitoring of the sleeping pulse rate, temperature, and ESR to assess the activity of the disease.
- Rheumatic fever and first diagnosis of rheumatic heart disease are both notifiable conditions.

Prophylaxis against recurrence:
- Penicillin until at least 21 years old.
- Benzathine penicillin IM monthly (dose 1,2 million units).
- Additional cover is necessary prior to dental procedures to prevent bacterial endocarditis. Amoxycillin by mouth one hour before dental treatment. Dose: under ten years 1,5 g, and over ten years 3 g.

Recurrences are common and are of great importance, as each new attack is likely to damage the heart still further.

Complications of rheumatic heart disease
- Congestive cardiac failure in the active or inactive phases.
- Damage to valves and endocardium resulting in one or more of the following:
  - Mitral incompetence (MI).
  - Mitral stenosis (MS).
  - Aortic incompetence (AI).

Parental information
The implications of the child's condition must be explained to the parents, especially the importance of prevention of streptococcal infections which may result in recurrence of the rheumatic disease and further cardiac damage. At the same time, they must not overprotect the child, or he or she may become a 'cardiac cripple' unnecessarily. For decisions regarding participation in sport, consult a cardiac clinic or other expert in heart disease.

Sydenham's chorea
This is a form of acute rheumatic fever and may be the only sign of the disease. It is characterised by the gradual onset of irregular, jerky, and unintentional movements of the face and limbs. The movements are

usually bilateral, although occasionally one-sided. They tend to get worse when the child is stressed and disappear during sleep. School teachers may complain that the child is inattentive in class and is clumsy, fidgety, and emotionally unstable, with frequent outbursts of crying. Girls are more often affected than boys (±3:1), and the onset is usually between five and 15 years. Children with this condition are often bright and intelligent.

Prognosis
A self-limiting disease, but may last for three to four months.

Action
Any suspected case should be referred to hospital for assessment.

Management
Refer for full assessment and further control, that is, Haloperidol (Serenace®) and penicillin.

Central nervous system

Behaviour disturbances and common 'pre-school' problems

Attention Deficit / Hyperactivity Disorder (ADHD)

Attention Deficit / Hyperactivity Disorder is the most commonly diagnosed behavioral disorder of childhood. It is estimated to affect from 3–5% of school-age children. It often has far-reaching negative effects on their social and emotional development as well as on their performance in school and future work settings. Symptoms cover a wide range of different behaviour, but these can be divided into the following categories:

1. **Poor attention**: The child is careless, inattentive, disobedient, disorganised, has poor concentration (daydreamer), and is absent-minded and forgetful.
2. **Impulsivity**: The child shows disruptive and impatient behaviour and interrupts regularly.
3. **Hyperactivity**: The child fidgets constantly, has a short attention span, and is noisy and excessively talkative.

If untreated, ADHD affects the child's education, social development, health, future work capability, the family unit's functioning, financial load, and health, especially with regards to the emotional burden. ADHD also has an effect on society. It is often associated with an increase in driving accidents as well as delinquent and criminal behaviour and drug abuse.

Correct diagnosis and treatment is critical. The appropriate use of drugs such as Ritalin® makes better management and education possible.

Attention-seeking behaviour

This includes dirt-eating, breaking of ornaments, pulling up flowers in the garden, shouting attacks, turning on taps, swearing, and innumerable other tricks which the child knows will cause anger and distress in the parent or guardian.

Wherever possible, such tricks should be ignored and the child should not be punished. What must be determined is why the child is behaving in this way to draw attention to him- or herself. This may be difficult to define and even more difficult to correct.

Breath-holding attacks

If an attack occurs only when the child is thwarted, as little fuss as possible must be made. On no account must the child be allowed to have his or her way as a result of the attack. Such attacks may be quite frightening to attendants, as prolonged breath-holding may even result in a convulsion and temporary unconsciousness. As soon as this occurs, breathing will recommence spontaneously, the child will wake up, and the attack will be over.

Breath-holding with convulsions must be distinguished from true epilepsy, which is usually followed by a post-ictal state of unconsciousness for some time after the fit is over.

Breath-holding attacks usually disappear by the age of five or six years, but when present, they are very difficult to prevent. Anti-convulsant drugs play no part in the management.

Not all breath-holding attacks are behaviour disorders. The type of attack which occurs only when the child is unexpectedly hurt, for instance after a sudden fall, is similar to a vasovagal attack and is in no way related to parental mismanagement.

Discipline

Three essential components are necessary for children to develop security in their young lives. These are love, discipline, and routine. Authority must be firm, kind, reasonable, and consistent. This results in a sense of security which is essential for a child's emotional development. On the other hand, excessive discipline is definitely harmful.

Together with discipline, punishment must be reasonable and consistent. It must not occur during a loss of temper, or during the stage where the parent's reaction is irrational because of anger. Remember that children are more likely to behave well because they want the approval of their parents or teacher, than because of fear of punishment. Praise and reward are better means of handling a situation than punishment. The spanking of a child should never be intended to inflict actual pain, but rather to convey intense disapproval of his or her actions. Spanking in certain circles is being viewed as a form of child abuse.

Left-handedness

If a child is consistently left-handed, no effort should be made to force them to use their right hand. If, however, they are ambidextrous, they should be encouraged to use the right hand, as long as they show no anxiety in this regard. We live in a right-hand orientated world which is not going to change.

Masturbation

From the age of about five months when a boy learns to grasp objects, he will also grasp his penis. This is completely normal and no attention need be paid to such exploratory manipulations.

True masturbation, however, may occur in fairly young children. This is usually done quite openly, unless the child has been punished for it; it is then practised in secret. On no account should any fuss be made about it. It is important to instruct parents in this matter, as undue attention and punishment create problems rather than the actual masturbation itself.

Nail-biting

Many children bite their nails and it is a harmless (if ugly) habit. Any cause of insecurity should be determined and removed if possible.

Punishment rarely succeeds in breaking the habit, and is more likely to make the situation worse. Support, encouragement, and understanding are more likely to be successful; parents could also try to reward the child for not biting his or her nails.

Negativism

Many children who are charming and react positively up to the age of 12 months suddenly become awkward and negative between the age of one and three years. They can then be expected to do the exact opposite of what they are asked to do.

This is a normal stage of ego development, and if the parents understand this and accept it with a sense of humour, no behaviour problem will develop. This stage must not become a battle of will between parents and child.

Pica

This is the abnormal desire to eat something which is different or strange and which would normally not be eaten, for example sand, charcoal, newspaper, etc. It is common in normal children up to the age of two years. After the age of two it may be an attention-seeking device associated with an emotional upset. It also occurs frequently in mentally challenged children.

There is a greater incidence of pica in children who have iron deficiency anaemia. Children with pica, in turn, also have an increased incidence of parasitic infestation, which may aggravate the anaemia. All children with pica must have a haemoglobin or full blood count done as part of the assessment and potential worm parasites should be treated.

Treatment depends on the cause. If it is being used as an attention-seeking device, the parents must not display anxiety or overreact on seeing the child eating dirt or other substances, as this is exactly the reaction the child is trying to create.

Potty-training

There is wide variation in the normal developmental pattern, but most children will tell their parents in sufficient time that they want to be placed on the potty by about two years of age. Training must be carried out with as little stress as possible, and it is usually best to wait until around two years of age before beginning training. At no stage should the child be punished for soiling clothes or bed linen, even when partially trained. Make this training period as pleasant and as much fun as possible. Reward systems work well with most children. Start with a potty on the ground, as toilets are frightening and awkward for a small child.

Stuttering

All children who stutter should be referred for full assessment and the necessary speech therapy. This can be a serious condition, and needs early professional intervention if it is not to become a lifelong problem.

Temper tantrums

Most children have at least one temper tantrum. If they attract attention, cause anxiety, or get their own way by having a tantrum, they soon realise that they can use it to get what they want and the tantrums continue. Immediate withdrawal of the parent / caregiver from the scene usually ends the tantrum. Children learn to manipulate their parent, and it is therefore best to ignore such tantrums. However, if well established, sources of insecurity, excessive strictness and so forth, must be found and corrected, if possible.

Thumb-sucking

All babies suck their thumbs, fingers, or a dummy at some stage. No treatment is required unless it continues beyond the age of six years, when it may cause deformity of the front teeth. It usually stops spontaneously if it is ignored, or if gentle loving persuasion is used. Thumb-sucking can be prolonged by insecurity.

Tics

Facial grimaces or blinking tics are very common and indicate an underlying anxiety condition. Determine the cause if possible, and manage accordingly with support, encouragement, and understanding.

CNS conditions

Bell's palsy

Idiopathic unilateral facial paralysis of sudden onset.

Cause unknown but presumed to be of viral origin. Swelling of seventh (facial) nerve causes ischaemia and subsequent paralysis.

Clinical features

- Affected side is smooth and free from wrinkles – expressionless.
- Dribbling of saliva out of affected side of mouth.
- Lower eyelid droops and the mouth angle sags on the affected side.
- Unable to close the eye tightly on the affected side.
- Pain behind the ear may precede the facial weakness.

Note: History of chronic ear infection or discharge needs urgent referral, as palsy may be secondary to middle ear infection.

Prognosis

Complete recovery within months in 90% of cases.

Treatment

Oral steroids may be of benefit if given early. Refer urgently for treatment.

Cerebral palsy (See pp. 72–75)

Collective term used for many different non-progressive neurological dysfunctions which cause a disturbance of posture or movement.

Predisposing factors

Brain damage in utero, during the perinatal period, or during the first two years of life. Fetal hypoxia during labour remains an important cause in under-resourced countries such as South Africa.

Presentation
- Delay in both fine and gross motor development.
- May have spasticity, involuntary movements, seizures, intellectual disability, visual or auditory defects as well.

Treatment
- Prevention: Good antenatal, labour, and neonatal care.
- Early detection and referral for plan of management and optimal physiotherapy.
- Comprehensive assessment and ongoing care in a specialised centre is ideal, but appropriate home care can be achieved with appropriate guidance.
- Ongoing support.

Concussion / head injury *(See Common surgical problems, p. 323)*

If, after a head injury, there is any evidence of memory loss, vomiting, convulsions, confusion, depressed level of consciousness, or drainage of blood or CSF from ear or nose, the child must be referred to hospital immediately.

If there was any loss of consciousness, no matter how brief, the child should also be referred for assessment. In other cases not referred, the parents must be warned to be alert for the onset of increasing drowsiness, headache, vomiting, undue irritability, incessant crying or loss of interest in eating, toys, and play. If any of these develop, the child should be referred immediately, as there may be intracranial bleeding. Ideally, this warning should be documented in the folder or clinic card.

Convulsions

These consist of abnormal movements with local or generalised jerking or spasm of muscles. Loss of consciousness is commonly associated with it. Before the convulsion starts, disturbances of sensation (an aura) or abnormal behaviour may occur. Convulsions may have tonic (patient stiff, tone is increased) or clonic (patient has jerking movements) aspects.

Other words used for convulsions are fits and seizures.

Causes
- **Primary:** The largest group; no detectable cause.
- **Secondary:** Due to CNS disease or injury, for example:
  - Meningitis or encephalitis.
  - Brain abscess.
  - Tumour.

- ○ Haemorrhage.
- ○ Brain injury.
- ○ Metabolic disorders, for example:
  - – Hypoglycaemia.
  - – Hypernatraemia.
  - – Hypoxia.
  - – Kernicterus (bilirubin encephalopathy).
- ○ Fever, six months to six years.
- ○ Hypertension, for example acute glomerulonephritis.
- ○ Poisons / toxins, for example:
  - – Insecticides.
  - – Lead (rare in South Africa).
- ○ Shigella infection.
- **Epilepsy:** Causes recurrent convulsions.

Clinical features of epilepsy
Grand mal
This consists of three phases:
- Aura (headache, irritability, abnormal behaviour, sensations or fears) may be present.
- Tonic phase.
- Clonic phase.

The fit may be local, unilateral or generalised. Localised twitching may progress to generalised fits. The child usually loses consciousness. It may be followed by a transient limb paralysis (Todd's Paresis), which may last from 24 hours to a few days. In the very young, seizures may only present as flickering of the eyes, or as apnoea.

Petit mal
Usually occurs from six years of age. It appears as a momentary loss of consciousness without abnormal movements. The child does not fall to the floor, and a vacant stare may be the only sign of a seizure. Often described as absence spells. These usually occur many times a day, and may interfere with school performance.

Temporal lobe
May manifest with abnormal behaviour, repetitive movements, smacking of lips, hallucinations of hearing and taste, uncontrollable laughter, or nocturnal screaming. Usually abrupt onset and ending. May also have mental disturbance, with short attention span and poor concentration ability.

Management of a convulsion
Immediate
- Maintain a clear airway by extending neck and pushing jaw forward.
- Prevent injury from sharp objects during convulsing phase.
- Do no attempt to force a gag between the teeth, as this often causes more damage than it prevents. The bitten tongue heals quickly.
- Give oxygen.
- Rectal diazepam (Valium®) 0,5mg per kilogram (use a small syringe); maximum 10 mg. Repeat after ten minutes if necessary.
- Check blood glucose and correct if necessary.
- Take blood pressure in case fit is due to hypertension.
- Reduce fever if present.
- Exclude underlying meningitis or raised intracranial pressure.

Later
- Refer child after first convulsion for investigation and management.
- Anticonvulsant therapy is usually started only after a second fit, and is usually continued for two years after last convulsion.
- Measurement of control is assessed by frequency of convulsions.
- Dosage and type of anticonvulsant is determined at secondary / tertiary care levels.

Indications for referring a patient on long-term management back to hospital are:
- Poor control of convulsions (compliance often a problem).
- Side effects of drugs.

Febrile convulsions
Convulsions may occur in young children during the phase of increasing fever from whatever cause. There is often a strong family history of febrile convulsions.

For a fit to be accepted as a febrile convulsion, it should be:
- Associated with fever (fever before not after convulsion).
- In a child aged between six months and six years (rare after six years).
- Generalised, that is, bilateral.
- Lasting no longer than five minutes.
- Not followed by residual paralysis (Todds' paresis).

Management

For management of the acute attack, see Management of convulsions, p. 132.

Prevention and advice to parents regarding further illness:
- Do not over-dress child.
- Tepid (lukewarm) sponge child with very high fever and 'fan' with towel to cool.
- Paracetamol (e.g. Panado®).
- Anti-convulsants may be prescribed after two or three such convulsive episodes.

Note: Refer for investigation and further treatment after the first convulsion.

Differential diagnosis
- Breath-holding attack (convulsions cease when breathing is resumed).
- Fainting (no associated convulsion).

Coma

Definition

Loss of consciousness with no response to any external stimulation, including pain. (Stupor is loss of consciousness with response to stimulation.)

Causes

There are many different causes. Some are:
- Overdose of drugs / sedatives / anticonvulsants.
- Poisoning / alcohol.
- Following a convulsion.
- Hypoglycaemia.
- Meningitis.
- Head injury.
- Liver failure.

Emergency management
- Maintain the airway by extending the neck and holding the jaw forward.
- Provide oxygen and bag-and-mask ventilation if needed.
- Check blood glucose and treat hypoglycaemia if present.
- Measure blood pressure.

- Look for a cause:
  - If patient vomits, keep for analysis, toxicology.
  - Put on urine bag for urine testing and analysis.
  - Refer to hospital urgently.

Bacterial meningitis (Acute)
This is a paediatric emergency.

Definition
Infection of the meninges by bacteria, either blood-born or from a neighbouring focus, for example the middle ear.

Aetiology
Newborn period:
- Organisms are often Gram-negative, for example *E coli*. Less commonly Gram-positive, for example streptococci.

Over age of two to three months:
- Pneumococcus.
- *Haemophilus influenzae* (current vaccine will prevent).
- Meningococcus.
- Tuberculosis.

In most cases, the organism enters the CSF through the blood, but infection may also result from:
- Skull fracture.
- Chronic otitis media, mastoiditis.
- Meningomyelocele.
- Focal tuberculoma in brain.

Clinical features
Newborn
- Specific signs such as neck stiffness or bulging fontanelle are usually absent.
- Infant 'not doing well'.
- Feeding poorly, vomiting, poor suck.
- Apathetic, hypotonic.
- Jaundice.
- Apnoea or cyanotic attacks.
- Often has signs of septicaemia, for example hypothermia, poor perfusion, oedema, etc.

Infants: some or all of the following
- Fretful or irritable.
- High fever.
- Poor feeding, frowning.
- High-pitched cry.
- Tense or bulging anterior fontanelle.
- Convulsions.
- Vomiting.
- Possibly neck stiffness.

Toddlers and older children
- Fever.
- Headache.
- Vomiting.
- Irritability.
- Photophobia.
- Full fontanelle (up to ± 18 months of age when fontanelle is usually closed).
- Neck stiffness.
- Positive Brudzinski sign.
- Positive Kernig sign.
- Convulsions.
- Opisthotonos (usually late).
- Altered level of consciousness or coma.

Management
Refer any suspected case to hospital immediately for lumbar puncture and blood culture. This is a very serious illness, especially in neonates. Do not wait until diagnosis is obvious, as this will be too late for successful treatment.
- If clinical diagnosis is made, antibiotics (IV Ceftriaxone, or Cefuroxime must be given if there is likely to be any delay in reaching hospital. Delay in starting treatment may be fatal.
- If convulsing, give rectal Valium® as for convulsions (see p. 132).
- A purpuric rash strongly suggests meningococcal infection and immediate treatment with IV penicillin is required.

Complications
- Subdural effusion.
- Hydrocephalus – rapid increase in head circumference, for example more than 0,5 cm per week; due to blocking of drainage of CSF.

- Convulsions.
- Mental and motor disability, blindness, deafness.
- Personality change.

Note: Follow up all patients after discharge for developmental assessment and hearing screen. Even those who appear normal may show defects later.

Prognosis
This depends on:
- Early clinical diagnosis.
- Early and adequate treatment.
- Accurate laboratory diagnosis (CSF examination).
- Age (worse for newborns).

In general, mortality rate is up to 50% in newborns and 6–10% in older children, even with early treatment.

Special cases
Meningococcal meningitis
May have a very rapid course and may be accompanied by meningococcal septicaemia. The typical purpuric rash appears early in the illness and, if untreated, the disease is rapidly fatal. It is therefore an absolute emergency. Such cases should not have a lumbar puncture because of associated cerebral oedema and the danger of coning. Antibiotic **(penicillin**, **cefotaxime** or **ceftriaxone)** treatment needs to be started immediately.

TB meningitis
The onset is often gradual with changes in behaviour and increased sleepiness. The meningeal signs may be less obvious than in acute bacterial meningitis. Early diagnosis and treatment are equally important. There may be early warning signs such as unexplained weight loss and apathy.

Viral meningitis
Aetiology
This includes:
- Mumps, measles, chicken pox.
- Coxsackie.

- Echo.
- Polio.

Clinical features
- As in bacterial meningitis, may have fever, vomiting, and headache, but child is not as toxic or as ill-looking.
- Headache which often improves following lumbar puncture (decreased pressure).
- Usually shows improvement within 48 hours.
- Diagnosis determined by lumbar puncture and laboratory examination of CSF. No organisms found on Gram stain or culture. Viral origin usually assumed, as viral culture of CSF not done routinely. 'Neighbourhood' causes and TB meningitis may confuse diagnosis. Often best to call such cases aseptic meningitis until certain of viral diagnosis.

Complications
Uncommon.

Management
- Control fever.
- Give oral fluids, or give IV at first if child is vomiting.
- If unsure, and especially if under-two-years age group, rather over-treat (with antibiotics) than under-treat.

Prognosis
Very good.

Note: As it is impossible to distinguish bacterial from viral meningitis without CSF examination, all cases must be referred.

Ear, nose, mouth, and throat

Coryza (The common cold)

Definition

An acute viral infection of the upper respiratory tract which involves the nasal airways. The sinuses and middle ear may also become involved in the process.

Epidemiology

It occurs mainly in:

- Young children who have older siblings, as the siblings are exposed to new viruses at school.
- In children from overcrowded homes.
- Those attending crèches.

Causative organisms

A wide variety of viruses.

Clinical features

- Fever for a few days.
- Clear mucoid discharge from the nose, often accompanied by a cough.
- A blocked nose which may interfere with feeding in young children.

Complications

The infection may spread to sinuses, the middle ear cavities, the larynx, and the bronchi. Bacterial secondary infection often follows and is recognised by the appearance of a purulent nasal discharge.

Management

- Anti-fever measures.
- No antibiotic is required unless secondary bacterial infection is present.
- Nose drops: Iliadin® drops, three times daily for two days. Use only if obstruction of upper airways interferes with feeding in small children.
- Decongestant, for example Actifed®, Demazin®.

Note: If the nasal discharge is unilateral, consider the possibility of a foreign body. If the nasal discharge is bloodstained, consider diphtheria. In an infant, consider congenital syphilis.

Epistaxis (Nose bleeding)

Bleeding most commonly occurs from the small blood vessels on the mucosa of the nasal septum. Many children will have a few brief nose bleeds and these should cause no undue concern. Repeated or severe nose bleeds, however, need attention.

Causes of repeated or severe nose bleeds may include:
- Allergic rhinitis: The nasal mucosa is chronically inflamed and bleeds very easily; this is the most common cause.
- Nose picking / local trauma.
- Foreign body in a nostril: The bleeding will be from the side with the foreign body.
- Blood diseases (bleeding tendency).
- Hypertension.
- Liver disease (bleeding tendency).
- Systemic infections, for example rheumatic fever.

Treatment

To stop a bleed, pinch the soft part of the nose so that the nasal septum is compressed for five to ten minutes. This procedure promotes clot formation. It may be necessary to repeat the measure a few times. Refer urgently if the bleeding is difficult to control.

Recurrent episodes of epistaxis need referral for investigation and cauterisation of bleeding areas.

Herpes stomatitis (See also Infectious diseases, p. 208)

This is an acute illness of young children associated with fever and painful mouth ulcers.

Epidemiology
- The common age is one to three years.
- The condition is often seen with measles and kwashiorkor, due to lowered cellular immunity.

Cause
- Primary infection with herpes simplex virus (mainly type I).
- Herpes simplex is the most common cause of ulcers in the mouth in children:

○ Type I: Mainly skin and mouth.
○ Type II: Genitalia.

Clinical features

- A sudden onset of fever over one to two days.
- The gums are commonly swollen and bleed easily.
- There is usually swelling of the submandibular lymph glands.
- Excessive salivation is very common.
- Small, blister-like lesions develop anywhere inside the mouth and on the tongue. These break down and then appear as greyish-yellow ulcers which later slough, leaving a red base. They are extremely painful for the first five or six days of the illness.
- Because of the pain, the infants feed poorly and salivate excessively.
- The breath is not foul-smelling.
- The disease is self-limiting over eight to ten days.
- Herpes and thrush often occur together in patients whose immunity is suppressed (e.g. HIV infection).

Management

- Anti-fever measures.
- Encourage oral fluids to avoid dehydration and make repeated reassessments of the child's state of hydration.
- Avoid hot or acid fluids which will cause pain. Bland fluids are best, especially lukewarm milk.
- Keep the mouth clean. Glycerine keeps the mouth moist. Teejel® may be of value, or the mouth may be washed with bicarbonate of soda solution.
- Hospitalisation for nasogastric feeds may be necessary.
- Antibiotics are of no use.
- Acyclovir is used in severe cases and in children with symptomatic HIV infection who have frequent recurrent episodes.

Complications requiring referral

- Dehydration as a result of poor intake.
- Herpetic lesions of the eye (herpetic keratitis), which may result in corneal ulceration and blindness.
- Herpetic vulvovaginitis or urethritis.
- Disseminated herpes, especially in newborn, malnourished or immunosuppressed children. A potentially fatal disease.

Note: Once a child has experienced a primary herpes infection, lesions may reappear on the outside of the lips (fever blisters) in association with respiratory infections, especially pneumococcal or other infections throughout life (secondary herpes).

Palatal defects (Cleft palate)

Congenital defects may involve the soft and / or hard palate, and vary in severity. They may also be associated with cleft lip. It is important to examine mouths of all newborn babies with a torch and spatula, paying special attention to the back of the palate.

Complications

Early

- Feeding difficulties which may result in failure to thrive.
- Recurrent respiratory tract infections due to inhalation of feeds and nasal regurgitation.
- Chronic otitis media from milk entering Eustachian tubes.

Late

- Speech defects.
- Hearing loss.
- Dental problems.
- Emotional problems.

Management

- The mother will require reassurance while she learns to feed the infant. Breastfeeding is the best method of feeding babies with palatal clefts. The areola is drawn into the mouth and effectively covers even quite large defects.
- Babies may be able to feed from a normal bottle and teat, especially if the hole is enlarged. Feeding with a teaspoon and cup is a good method in cases with a large cleft.
- The infant should be referred to a hospital where facilities are available for surgical repair, orthodontic treatment, and speech therapy. Referral in the first month of life will enable the best time for surgery to be decided.

Thrush

A common yeast infection of the mouth, gastrointestinal tract or nappy area in the young infant or immunocomprised child.

Epidemiology

There are four groups at risk:

- The newborn and / or very young infant. Thrush frequently affects newborn babies, who may acquire the infection during delivery, from their mother's nipples or from unsterile bottle teats.
- Children with kwashiorkor.
- Children with measles.
- Children with immune deficiency, for example HIV.

Note: In all of these situations, there is a degree of lowered cellular immunity.

Causative organism

The yeast fungus *Candida albicans*.

Clinical features

- White plaques which look like deposits of milk occur on mucous membranes of mouth and tongue.
- Mild thrush is common and asymptomatic and does not interfere with feeding.
- White, raised, ulcer-like areas, which may also resemble milk curds. If scraped, the lesions bleed, whereas milk deposits will not bleed.
- Poor feeding is a common feature of severe thrush.
- The perineum, if involved, is red and excoriated (raw), with additional discrete yellowish macules. Perineal thrush does not respond to ordinary nappy rash treatment. Thrush occurs in creases while nappy rash is worse on exposed areas.

Complications

- Dehydration due to poor feeding: Try cup and spoon feeding.
- Secondary infection.
- Systemic complications (only in children with reduced immunity).

Management

Prevention

- Improve bottle hygiene.
- Improve the child's nutritional state.
- If the baby is bottlefed, boil the bottles and teats, as Milton® or Jik® are ineffective against monilia. Dummies must also be boiled or be discarded.

Treatment
- Mycostatin® suspension 1 ml dropped into the mouth after feeds, or Mycostatin® ointment rubbed on to the oral membrane (less expensive and more effective).
- Mycostatin® ointment is also used on nappy area.

Treat thrush if present in mother with:
- Mycostatin® cream for nipples.
- Pessaries for vaginal thrush.

Acute tonsillitis

Definition
Infection of the tonsils and pharynx.

Epidemiology
- May occur at any age.
- Transmission is by droplet spread.
- If there is recurrent streptococcal infection, there is often a carrier in the family.

Aetiology
- 90% are caused by viruses.
- Beta-haemolytic streptococcus cause most of the other cases.

Clinical features
Some or all of the following may be present:
- The child may look ill and flushed.
- Fever.
- Sore throat.
- Poor feeding.
- Earache due to referred pain or otitis media.
- Vomiting.
- Red pharynx and tonsils.
- Follicular tonsillitis (exudate confined to tonsillar fossae).
- Cervical lymph glands enlarged and tender.
- Meningism: Neck stiffness (often misdiagnosed as meningitis).

Differential diagnosis
- Infectious mononucleosis.
- Diphtheria: The membrane may extend beyond the tonsillar area.

Management (See Indications for tonsillectomy, p. 146)

General
- Anti-fever measures.
- Avoid dehydration by giving extra fluids by mouth.

Specific
- Antibiotics: Oral penicillin V or amoxicillin for 14 days.

Note: As it is impossible to differentiate clinically between viral and streptococcal tonsillitis, it is wise to treat all patients with penicillin in order to avoid the possible complications of rheumatic fever and acute nephritis in untreated cases of streptococcal infection.

A possible exception is the young child or infant with other signs of viral upper respiratory tract infection, for example coryza. The danger of rheumatic fever developing is greater in the child over three years.

Refer
- If a membrane is present.
- If fever persists for more than 48 hours on treatment.

Complications
- Acute otitis media.
- Peritonsillar abscess (quinsy) which is a large swelling above one or both tonsils.
- Acute nephritis occurring two or three weeks after throat infection.
- Acute rheumatic fever infection two or three weeks later.

Tonsillar membrane
Definition
A sheet-like membrane firmly attached to the tonsils and / or posterior pharyngeal wall, which will bleed when scraped. The colour may be grey, white or even black.

Causes
There are several possible causes, which include:
- Diphtheria.
- Infectious mononucleosis.
- Agranulocytosis (low granulocyte count in the blood).
- Severe tonsillitis (confined to tonsillar fossae).

- Post-tonsillectomy slough: This can look very like diphtheria, but the spread is not beyond the operation site.
- Corrosive (acid and alkali) burns.

Referral
All cases should be referred unless it is certain that the lesion is a post-tonsillectomy slough.

Peritonsillar abscess (Quinsy)
An acute infection extending into the tissues behind the tonsil and superior constrictor muscle; usually an extension of infection from tonsil.

Causative organism
Usually group A beta-haemolytic Streptococcus.

Clinical features
- The child is febrile and toxic.
- There is severe pain on swallowing.
- The head is held tilted towards affected side.
- There may be marked trismus (difficulty in opening jaw).
- The child will often dribble saliva.

Treatment
- Refer to hospital.
- The quinsy may need incision and drainage.
- See Indications for tonsillectomy below.

Indications for tonsillectomy
- Four or more episodes of tonsillitis in preceding 12 months.
- Peritonsillar abscess (quinsy).
- Unilateral tonsillar enlargement (tumour).
- Obstructive sleep apnoea syndrome.
- Recurrent or persistent streptococcal pharyngeal infections.
- Chronic non-specific infection of the tonsils.
- Recurrent or persistent cervical lymphadenitis.
- Tuberculous cervical lymphadenitis.

Adenoidal hypertrophy
This is marked enlargement of the adenoids, which results in a relative narrowing of the upper airway and resulting interference with the drainage of the middle ear *via* the Eustachian tube.

Clinical features
• Mouth breathing.
• Nasal speech.
• Frequent snoring at night which may wake the child from sleep.
• Recurrent otitis media.
• Post-nasal discharge causing cough at night with rhino-bronchitis.

Indications for adenoidectomy
• Three or more episodes of acute otitis media in preceding 12 months.
• Chronic secretory otitis media.
• Obstructive sleep apnoea syndrome.
• Two or more of the following:
  ○ Mouth breathing.
  ○ Snoring.
  ○ Recurrent sinusitis.
• All children undergoing tonsillectomy.

Snoring

Loud snoring during sleep is abnormal in childhood. Drowsiness, irritability, learning problems or poor school performance, enuresis, chest deformity, and pulmonary hypertension may all occur as a result of obstructed breathing during sleep. The patient should be referred for adenoidectomy.

Wax in the ear (Cerumen)

This is a normal secretion of ceruminous glands situated in the outer part of the external meatus. It has powerful anti-bacterial and anti-fungal properties, and is necessary for the normal health of the external auditory canal. The quantity, quality, and colour of wax vary in different people.

Clinical features
If large quantities of wax accumulate or become hard, partial deafness may result.

Treatment
Syringe the ear. This should only be done if the canal is completely obstructed, causing partial deafness.

Note
• Before syringing, check for a history of discharge. If there is a possibility of a dry perforation, do not syringe.

- Inspection: If wax is hard, first soften it with warm olive oil inserted into canal twice daily, or Cerumenex® 30 minutes to one hour before syringing.

Method of ear syringing
- A metal syringe is easily controlled. Make sure the plunger slides easily and nozzle is screwed on firmly.
- Use tap water at 37 °C to avoid vertigo (giddiness).
- Direct the stream of water along roof of external ear canal and avoid excessive force, which may cause a perforation.
- Dry canal well, as a moist ear may lead to otitis externa.
- Inspect ear drum for perforation. Syringing ear will result in pink drum immediately afterwards; of no significance.
- If unable to remove wax with syringe, refer.

Foreign body in the ear
A variety of objects find their way into the external auditory canals of children, for example beads, pips, etc. Clumsy removal of an object may rupture the tympanic membrane. Try gently syringing the ear with lukewarm water first; if the object is not dislodged, the child should be referred to a specialist to have it removed.

Live objects, particularly insects, are very distressing to young children because of their buzzing and fluttering. Kill the insect by inserting olive / vegetable oil, and then remove by syringing the ear. Filling the ear with any harmless fluid, even water, will cause most insects to float upwards, so that they can be removed with forceps.

Otitis externa
This is an inflammation of the outer ear canal which occurs quite commonly in children, particularly in swimmers.

Causes
- Crowded swimming pools are a frequent source of infection. Failure to dry ears well after bathing may be a contributing factor.
- Children with eczema are more likely to develop otitis externa.
- Trauma caused by scratching the canal or by insertion of a foreign body, may result in infection.

Clinical features
- The ear is painful, and this is made worse by movement of the pinna, or by pressure on the tragus and opening of mouth.

- The outer ear canal is red and swollen.
- A scanty discharge, which may be serous or purulent.
- Deafness if the external canal is blocked.
- Painful, enlarged lymph nodes may be felt around pinna.
- A boil (furuncle) may develop in the meatal wall.

Treatment
- Ear cleaning: Removal of all debris with cotton wool on an orange stick. The cotton wool must project beyond the stick, or the drum may be injured.
- Insert local antibiotic drops, for example Chloramphenicol, Soframycin®, Polymixin® three times daily.
- If a furuncle (boil) is present, it will require analgesics, systemic antibiotic treatment, and may need surgical drainage.
- Super-added fungal infection may require treatment.

Prevention and advice
- No swimming during the acute stage.
- Do not scratch the ears.
- Remove all debris regularly with an orange stick and cotton wool.
- Stop use of drops when better.
- Treat eczema in other areas of the body if present.

Acute otitis media
An acute infection of the middle ear mostly bacterial, sometimes viral.

Aetiology
The causative organisms include a variety of bacteria:
- Streptococcus.
- Staphylococcus.
- Pneumococcus.
- *Haemophilus influenzae*: More common in children under two years of age.
- Bacterial infection often follows a viral upper respiratory tract infection.

Clinical features
- Fever.
- Earache: The child may rub or pull on the ear.
- Irritability and / or screaming attacks.
- Diarrhoea and vomiting may occur.

- Deafness.
- Pus may discharge from the ear once the ear drum has perforated.

On examination, the tympanic membrane varies in appearance at different stages:
- It loses its glistening character and the reflected cone of light is absent.
- It then becomes pink with dilation of vessels running over it and later appears red and bulging.
- Finally, the membrane perforates with a muco-purulent discharge from the ear.

Note: Pain diminishes when the drum perforates and mother may not seek medical help, as the child often stops complaining. Delay in treatment then results in additional complications such as:
- Mastoiditis.
- Destruction of middle ear ossicles leading to deafness.
- Intracranial infection, for example meningitis or brain abscess.
- Facial palsy (seventh cranial nerve).

Management
In the early stages
- Anti-fever measures.
- Analgesics.
- Decongestants, for example Iliadin® or Drixine® drops to the nose for three days.
- Antibiotics: Co-trimoxazole or amoxicillin for ten days.

Later in the illness
- If the tymphanic membrane is bulging, refer patient for myringotomy (surgical incision of ear drum).
- If the drum has recently perforated and the ear is discharging:
  - Clean ear twice daily with cotton wool on an orange stick.
  - Antibiotic (as above).
  - If there is no improvement, send an ear swab to laboratory and change the antibiotic, depending on growth and the antibiotic sensitivity of organism.
  - Refer.

Differential diagnosis
- Toothache, due to pain being referred from the teeth to the ear.
- Mumps which presents as earache, but with normal eardrum.

- Otitis externa: Here the ear is tender if the tragus is pushed on.
- Foreign body in ear canal. This is seen on inspection with auroscope.

Chronic otorrhoea (Running ear)

A chronic discharging ear is of importance because it may lead to deafness, or to an intracranial infection.

Causes

- Chronic otitis externa.
- Chronic otitis media.
- A foreign body in the canal.

Treatment

- The mainstay is frequent dry mopping of the ear. The mother needs to be shown how deep to mop the ear three or four times a day. Use an orange stick with the tip covered with cotton wool. Commercial ear buds are usually too large to be effective.
- Decongestants such as Demazin®, Actifed®, Dimetapp®.
- Amoxicillin or co-trimoxazole orally.

Note: Diphtheria organisms may sometimes be cultured from a chronic discharging ear. Pus swabs are often not useful because of marked secondary contamination with non-pathogenic organisms. Tuberculosis is a rare cause of chronic resistant otitis media and is often associated with a facial nerve palsy on the side of the discharging ear.

Perforation of ear drum *(See figure 1.6, p.15)*

Before examining for a perforation, clean out the ear if necessary.

Central perforation

- This is usually safe and can be treated by frequent ear mopping, decongestants, and systemic antibiotics.
- Healing should occur, but may take several weeks.

Attic perforation (i.e. high up on tympanic membrane)

This is usually associated with mastoid air cell infection (mastoiditis), so refer as soon as possible as serious complications may result.

Referral

An ear that does not become dry after two weeks' treatment, or a perforation that does not heal in a month, should be referred for an ENT opinion.

Deafness

Normally, speech is learnt by hearing sounds. Children who do not hear speech in the first five years of life usually never learn to speak. For this reason, early diagnosis of hearing loss is essential for successful treatment and proper development of speech. It is therefore desirable to screen all babies for hearing loss at seven to nine months, using the rattle test.

Mothers are often the first people to realise their child is deaf, so their complaints must always be taken seriously.

Some of the ways in which hearing loss in infancy may present include:
- Failure to waken or respond to loud sounds.
- Parental concern that the baby does not hear.
- A baby who babbles normally at six months, but becomes much quieter at nine to ten months.

Methods of screening hearing
Small children
It is essential to use the proper acoustic rattle, which is usually available from the ENT departments of academic hospitals in the larger centres. The child sits facing forward on the mother's lap. The room must be quiet. The examiner stands behind the mother out of sight of the child. The rattle is held about 5 cm from the ear, and then turned through 90°. This will produce a soft, high-frequency sound. If the child can hear it, he or she will usually turn his or her head to look at the source of the sound. The other ear is then tested. If the result is doubtful, refer the child for formal audiometry at the ENT department of a suitably equipped hospital.

Older children
The easiest screening method is to stand behind the child and get him or her to repeat words that have been spoken (not whispered) into each ear at close range (10 cm). The Stycar screening tests are very useful when screening is done on a large scale. These require some simple special equipment.

Children particularly 'at risk' for hearing loss
- Family history of deafness.
- Maternal infections during pregnancy:
  ○ Rubella.
  ○ Cytomegalovirus infection.
- Prenatal conditions:

- o Very low birth weight (below 1500 g).
- o Severe fetal hypoxia.
- Postnatal:
  - o Congenital abnormalities of the external ear.
  - o Severe neonatal jaundice.
  - o Meningitis or encephalitis.
  - o Exposure to high doses of ototoxic drugs, for example gentamicin.
  - o Children who have had chronic / recurrent middle ear infections.

Causes of congenital and neonatal deafness

- Malformation of cochlear nerve.
- Intrauterine damage to cochlear nerve, for example following maternal rubella in first trimester.
- Severe fetal hypoxia.
- Marked immaturity.
- Severe neonatal jaundice.

Causes of acquired deafness (Late deafness)

- Blockage of external meatus by wax or a foreign body. If, after removal of wax or foreign body, deafness persists, refer.
- Otitis media.
- Meningitis or encephalitis.
- Mumps.
- Trauma to eighth nerve.
- Toxic action of drugs, for example streptomycin, gentamicin.

Prevention

- Genetic counselling.
- Good perinatal care, including the avoidance of hyper-bilirubinaemia.
- Immunisation against mumps and rubella.
- Monitoring of ototoxic drugs, for example gentamicin, streptomycin.
- Early diagnosis and adequate treatment of meningitis.
- Adequate treatment of chronic otitis media and chronic perforation.
- Avoidance of sudden loud noises, for example firecrackers.
- Monitor high decibel working areas.
- Wearing of protective ear muffs.

Teeth

Tooth development begins in utero. Calcification of deciduous teeth occurs within five months of gestation, and shortly after birth in the case of permanent teeth. There are two sets of teeth:

- **Temporary** or **milk teeth** (primary dentition) which start erupting from about six months of age; the complete dentition (20 teeth) is present by about two years.
- **Permanent teeth** (secondary dentition) which start erupting from five to six years (total number 32).

Table 7.1

Deciduous (20)	Usual age of eruption
Lower central incisors (2)	6–8 months
Upper central incisors (2)	7–9 months
Lower and upper lateral incisors (2 + 2)	8–11 months
Anterior molars (4)	10–16 months
Canines (4)	16–20 months
Posterior molars (4)	20–30 months
Permanent (32)	
First molar (4)	5–6 years
Incisors	6–9 years
Bicuspids (8)	9–12 years
Canines (4)	9–12 years
Second molars (4)	12–13 years
Third molars (4)	17–22 years

Teething

Many quite severe symptoms are wrongly ascribed to teething. The dangerous result of this can be that the symptoms and signs of serious illness, such as urinary tract infection or even meningitis, are ignored. Few of the symptoms ascribed to teething, such as fever, are in fact due to teething alone.

Teething causes the following symptoms:
- Increased salivation.
- Slight irritability.

- Local tenderness with poor eating.
- Slightly loose stools (never dehydration).

Note: No treatment is necessary.

Dental caries

Food particles, bacteria, and salivary deposits combine to form a substance known as plaque. This rapidly forms and settles around the base of the teeth and in the crevices. Bacteria act on the carbohydrate in plaque to form an acid. This acid attacks and wears away the tooth surface (enamel) and caries (decay) follows. Dental caries are the most common form of infection in humans.

Prevention of caries

- Fluoride 1 mg/day to pregnant mother (often given with iron).
- Fluoride preparations from birth to adolescence, unless the water is already fluorinated; toothpaste containing fluoride.
- Dental hygiene: Clean teeth regularly and thoroughly after eating.
- Correct diet: Avoid refined carbohydrates, for example sugar and sweets, as far as possible. If sweets are given, do so after meals.
- Regular visits to dentist.

Other dental problems, for example malocclusion, require early referral for treatment.

Regular dental hygiene is especially important in children with heart disease, as dental sepsis may result in bacterial infection of the heart valves. Dental treatment in these children must take place under additional penicillin cover.

Tetracycline should never be given to children under seven years of age, as it may cause permanent yellow discolouration of teeth enamel.

Chapter 8

Gastrointestinal system

Abdominal distension: Chronic
- Long-standing distension or swelling of the abdomen is a more common problem than acute abdominal distension.
- Toddlers between two and three years of age stand with their abdomens protruding; parents may think this is abnormal. This is merely due to the posture, with a lumbar lordosis.
- Children with kwashiorkor frequently have painless abdominal distension from a combination of liver enlargement and lax abdominal muscles.
- Severe constipation, Hirschsprung's disease, and rickets may all present with abdominal distension, which is usually painless.
- Common causes are flatus, fluid, faeces, fat, food, and other organs or masses.

Examine the abdomen carefully for:
- Enlarged liver (malnutrition, heart failure, metabolic disease, hepatitis, chirrhosis, HIV).
- Enlarged spleen (may be very large); portal hypertension or other, for example haemolytic anaemia.
- Masses, especially in the flank (Wilm's tumour of the kidney).
- Faecal masses.
- Distended loops of bowel (gaseous or fluid).
- Ascites (free fluid).
- Fetus: If pregnancy is suspected, do a pregnancy test.

For all these conditions, the child needs to be referred to hospital for investigation.

If the distension is thought to be secondary to malnutrition, no abnormal masses or organs will be found in the abdomen, apart from moderate liver enlargement, and there will be no history of constipation. Advise on the treatment of malnutrition and re-examine the child in a week or two.

Abdominal pain and distention (Including acute abdomen)
See Common surgical problems, p. 305.

Appetite: Poor

A poor appetite in a child who is otherwise well and gaining weight normally does not call for investigation and treatment. Loss of appetite associated with illness is dealt with by treating the primary cause.

Main causes for loss of appetite, apart from illness, are:
- A small child who needs less food than is being offered.
- The normal stage of negativism between one and three years where, as the ego develops, food refusal occurs; this must not become a 'battle of wills'.
- Giving snacks such as sweets, potato crisps, and cool drinks between meals, which then leads to food refusal at mealtimes.
- Force-feeding children: This conditions them to experience mealtimes as unpleasant and aggravates the situation. It must be emphasised to parents that it is never necessary to force a healthy child to eat. The effort to do so may lead to further food refusal, and aggravate rather than solve the problem.

Blood in stool

Fresh blood

On the outside of the stool – may be due to:
- **Anal fissure** usually associated with constipation (hard stool and pain on passing stools).
- Rectal or large bowel **polyps or tumours** may present with large amounts of fresh blood on the stool.

Mixed with the stool (with or without diarrhoea) – may be due to:
- **Parasites:** Especially *Trichuris trichuria* (whipworm) or amoebiasis.
- **Colitis** (usually with mucus), caused by shigella, the excess use of purgatives or enemas, inflammatory causes or amoebiasis.
- **'Redcurrant jelly'** (mucus and blood with little or no stool): Intussusception (usually in infants).

Altered blood (Melaena)

Such blood looks brown / black and has been partly 'digested' (altered by acid and enzymes), which indicates that it comes from the upper GIT, for example hiatus hernia, oesophagus (varices), stomach (acute erosions or ulcers), duodenal ulcers. It may also be due to blood that has been swallowed, for example from an epistaxis. Refer all cases of malaena to hospital for further investigations.

Note: Iron therapy causes grey, dull stools (they are not shiny, smelly, sticky, and tarry as in melaena).

Newborn (Blood in stool)

This may be due to:

- Swallowing of maternal blood during delivery
- Haemorrhagic disease of the newborn (vitamin K deficiency), with a bleeding tendency.

Occult blood

Such blood cannot be seen with the naked eye, and is microscopic. The constant loss may lead to severe anaemia, which may, in fact, be the presenting problem.

It is important to consider occult blood loss from the gut in any case of anaemia not responding as expected to treatment. Causes are oesophageal varices, ulcers, *Trichuris trichiura* (whipworm), and (rarely) cow's milk allergy.

Any general bleeding disorder may present with blood in the stools. If no obvious causes (such as parasites or anal fissures) are found, refer to doctor for special investigations.

Certain dietary intake or drugs, for example penicillin V, etc. may cause red dye discolouration of the stool. The following tests distinguish between dyes and blood.

Test 1: Haematest tablets: Positive test gives a blue discolouration of test paper around tablet, which indicates that blood is present.

Test 2: If no Haematest tablets are available, mix stool with water and use a urine reagent strip to test for blood.

Colic

Screaming attacks may occur in otherwise well and thriving babies during the first two or three months of life, usually in the late afternoons and evenings, and are common. They are extremely upsetting and stressful to parents, who may feel inadequate and guilty because they cannot get their baby to stop screaming. If the crying stops when the baby is picked up, it is not due to colic. The cause of colic is poorly understood. Attacks of 'colic' occur less commonly in children who are carried around on their mother's back. The condition is self-limiting; reassure parents of the benign nature of the condition.

Constipation

Mothers often feel that a healthy child must pass a stool every day. Breastfed infants may have a stool after each feed (five to six times a day), or one every four to five days and yet be normal. What is important is that the stools are of normal consistency.

Constipation is the infrequent passage of hard stools. It may present with soiling due to overflow and fermentation of stool around the impacted faces.

Faecal loading is the incomplete evacuation of stools (often of normal consistency), which results in faecal build-up.

Causes

- Acute **constipation** with abdominal distension and vomiting can be caused by intestinal obstruction. Refer to hospital.
- Anal **fissures**. Defecation is painful. This is diagnosed by inspection of the anal margin and blood streaking of the stool.
- **Poor intake** of dietary **fibre**.
- **Lack of adequate fluid intake** during hot weather, or in children who are pyrexial. Advise the mother to give extra water between meals. More common in bottle-fed than in breastfed infants.
- **Hirschsprung's disease**. An uncommon condition. Constipation is severe and associated with marked distension of the abdomen. The rectum will be empty on digital examination. Refer to hospital for investigation and rectal biopsy.
- Any **condition causing vomiting** and fluid loss may lead to mild constipation through lack of food passing through the intestine.
- **Pica**. Eating of sand, pebbles, etc. may cause constipation and / or anal fissure.
- Severe, chronic constipation associated with mismanagement of toilet training which leads to acquired **mega-colon**, is also occasionally seen. Fortunately it appears to be rare in African children. If it does occur, refer to hospital for establishment of normal bowel habit and to exclude other underlying pathology.

Treatment

Refer to hospital if Hirschsprung's disease or an acute surgical emergency is suspected. For the average child with constipation, extra fluids between meals and additional fibre, vegetables, or fruit are all that is necessary. If the baby is bottle-fed, try increasing the sugar content and giving extra water between feeds. Regular small doses of milk of magnesia (one teaspoon three times a day) for three to six days will often help to re-establish a normal bowel habit.

In the older child, increase the fibre content of the diet by giving high-fibre cereals, brown or whole-wheat bread, bran added to porridge, baked beans, dried fruit, etc.

If there is no improvement with these measures, give sorbitol or lactulose 5–15 ml eight-hourly and use a bowel stimulant such as Senokot® or Dulcolax® for one week. Do not use these strong laxatives for longer than this period. Refer to hospital if bowel action not corrected after one week's treatment.

Chronic long-standing constipation (months or years) is best referred to a centre experienced in dealing with this difficult problem, which will need long-term dietary and toilet training with stimulants, fibre, etc.

Diarrhoeal diseases

Definition

These are caused by a disturbance in the balance between the mechanisms controlling secretion and absorption of water and electrolytes in the intestine, which results in excessive loss of these in the stools. They are characterised by frequent, watery, unformed stools. Ask about the number and character of stools rather than enquire whether a child has diarrhoea, as interpretation as to what diarrhoea actually is varies widely.

In well-nourished children, diarrhoea tends to be self-limiting with hardly any morbidity or mortality. In malnourished or very young infants, recurrent or chronic diarrhoea occurs more commonly and is associated with an appreciable mortality.

Chronic or recurrent diarrhoea with or without signs of malabsorption requires specific investigation, as it may be due to less common diseases, such as cystic fibrosis or coeliac disease.

Repeated episodes of diarrhoea could be due to HIV/AIDS.

Acute infantile gastroenteritis

Influencing factors

- Age: Majority of cases are aged under one year.
- Nutrition: Increased incidence in undernourished infants.
- Breastfeeding reduces incidence.
- Socio-economic: Cycle of poverty and ignorance.
- Environment: Food / water supply.
- Sanitation: Hand-washing / feeding bottles.

- Cross-infection and chronicity / increased recurrence.
- Availability of treatment.
- HIV/AIDS could be a contributing factor.

Common causes
- **Non-specific**
  - Majority of cases. Cause uncertain. Presumed viral.
- **Viral**
  - Approximately 40% of winter diarrhoea. Rota virus.
- **Bacterial**
  - Approximately 20%; includes Salmonella, Shigella, Campylobacter, and pathogenic *E. coli*.
- **Parasitic**
  - *Entamoeba histolytica* (amoebiasis), Cryptosporidium (in HIV), *Giardia lamblia, Trichuris trichiura*. Seldom dehydrating.
- **Dietary**
  - Secondary lactose intolerance. This is an important cause of persistent diarrhoea, especially in malnourished children.
  - Cow's milk protein intolerance. Much less common. Diarrhoea and vomiting should follow the smallest amounts of food containing milk products, and should cease on withdrawal. Repeated challenge or refer for biopsy for confirmation.
- **Parenteral**
  - Many children presenting with diarrhoea may also have a parenteral disease which requires treatment, for example otitis media, respiratory or urinary tract infection.

Other less common causes of diarrhoea
- Coeliac disease.
- Cystic fibrosis.
- Malabsorption syndromes.
- Antibiotics.
- Food poisoning.

Complications of diarrhoea
Dehydration
As the intravascular compartment is maintained at all costs, fluid loss occurs from interstitial and intracellular fluid. Assessment is based on the state of the eyes, mouth, skin turgor, fontanelle, peripheral circulation, and blood pressure.

Assessment of degree of dehydration

Early signs
- Decreased skin turgor (loss of normal elasticity).
- Sunken eyes and fontanelle (infants).
- Thirst (increased).
- Urine output decreased (can only be accurately assessed if urine bag is used).
- Weight loss (if previous weight is known).

Following signs
- Pulse rate increases.
- Child has a poor peripheral circulation (compensatory shutdown).
- Apathetic and drinks poorly or not at all.

Late and final signs
- Blood pressure drops.
- Pulse is rapid and feeble.
- Poor perfusion of organs, especially kidney / brain.
- Decreased level of consciousness.
- Acidosis increases and death occurs.

Grading of dehydration

1. Potential dehydration: No signs are clinically apparent, but you are worried about the patient's condition because of severity of diarrhoea or vomiting.
2. When early signs are present, arbitrarily assessed as 5% dehydration.
3. When marked signs are present, arbitrarily assessed as 10% dehydration.
4. Shock: (Hypovolaemia)
   - Compensated: Blood pressure is still maintained.
   - Uncompensated: Blood pressure falls.

Shock

There is inadequate circulating intravascular volume, shown by tachycardia, a small pulse volume, poor peripheral circulation (capillary filling time normally less than four seconds), and later a fall in blood pressure. The last is a late and ominous sign. Capillary filling time is assessed by pressing on the sole of the foot with a finger and then counting in seconds how long it takes for the blanched area to regain its colour. The result of shock is poor perfusion of organs and tissue with poor oxygen and nutrient supply.

Immediate and rapid volume replacement is needed, whether blood pressure is normal (compensated shock) or has fallen (uncompensated shock).

Acidosis

Classically shown by deep sighing respiration, but in young infants may be seen as tachypnoea. Acidosis due to bircarbonate loss in the stools, poor tissue blood supply, poor renal blood flow, ketonaemia secondary to starvation and the ill-advised giving of medications, especially aspirin. Mild to moderate acidosis will be corrected by ordinary rehydration. If pH is less than 7,1, special treatment is required (see Fluid therapy, p. 168).

Electrolyte disturbances

See Fluid therapy, p. 168.

Ileus (See Common surgical problems, p. 306)

- The abdomen is distended and relatively silent on auscultation.
- Associated with severe infection, toxaemia or hypokalaemia.
- Exclude a surgical cause, for example volvulus or intussuscepion. Refer if uncertain or if associated with abdominal pain or bile-stained vomiting.
- Hypokalaemia must be corrected (see Fluid therapy, p. 168).

Vomiting

If bile-stained or persistent, refer for investigation of a possible surgical cause (i.e. obstruction).

Hypoglycaemia

This may occur, especially in malnourished children, even if receiving dextrose-containing oral or IV fluids. May present as jitteriness or a full convulsion. Test for hypoglycaemia and, if present, give extra oral sugar solution or IV glucose.

Convulsions

Clear airway and give oxygen; stop convulsions with rectal diazepam (Valium®). Check for treatable cause such as fever or hypoglycaemia. Give an oral loading dose of phenobarbitone to prevent further convulsions. Refer for investigation, as this may be due to other causes such as meningitis, cerebral vein thrombosis or electrolyte disturbance.

Treatment of diarrhoea
General measures
Mild diarrhoea
- Not dehydrated and not vomiting. Diarrhoea only. Usually well-nourished children.
- Continue normal milk or breastfeeds.
- Additional oral fluids usually sufficient, given as oral half-strength dextrose-Darrows solution ($1/2$ DD) or other oral rehydration solution (ORS) containing electrolyte and sugar for 24 hours.
  Salt Sugar Solution (SSS) can be used.
  Care-giver counselled to make up ORS and SSS.
- Check hydration next day. Warn parents of potential danger signs. Patient to return sooner if these occur.

Moderate diarrhoea
- Mildly dehydrated and vomiting.
- Replace bottle milk feeds with oral clear fluids for 12 hours. Then start milk feeds again. Continue breastfeeding with additional clear fluid as required.
- Maintenance or restoration of normal hydration with frequent reassessment of progress. This is most important.
- Potassium chloride 0,5 g orally three times daily for two to three days.
- Give an electrolyte and sugar solution, for example half-strength Darrows in 5% dextrose by mouth or ORS. Prolonged periods of clear fluids or diluted milk feeds must be avoided, especially in malnourished children. If hydration does not improve, or if vomiting is an ongoing problem, then continuous nasogastric or IV fluids are required.
- In an emergency: If no electrolyte solution is available, give the following SSS freely and frequently by mouth. One cup for every stool or as much as child will take (minimum 200 ml/kg/24 hours):
  1 litre of clean water; if in doubt, boil the water.
  Salt – half of a level 5 ml teaspoon or 5 ml measure.
  Sugar – eight level 5 ml teaspoons or 5 ml measures (or glucose if available).
  Don't persist with the above if improvement not rapidly evident.
- If ORS sachet available: Dissolve 1 sachet in a litre of clean water. If in doubt, boil the water.

Table 8.1 Fluid therapy in diarrhoeal disease

Condition	Type of fluid / route	Volume	Feeding
Not dehydrated			
Not dehydrated Not vomiting	Oral rehydration solution (ORS)	Per loose stool: Under two years: 100 ml Over two years: 200 ml	Continue breast- / bottle feeds
Not dehydrated But vomiting	ORS	Trial of oral rehydration as above. Reassess progress. NGT continuous feed or IV if vomiting severe	Continue breast- / bottle feeds; Pelargon® is a suitable milk
Dehydration: as assessed by drinking (thirst), eyes, fontanelle, and skin turgor			
5% dehydrated (Mild)	½ DD by NGT (naso-gastric tube)	1. Rehydration: 50 ml/kg 2. Ongoing losses: 30 ml/kg Reassess: IV if severe vomiting.	Nil per mouth (NPM) for six hours. Then feed as above. If milk vomited, give ORS.
10% dehydrated (Moderate)	½ DD by IV	1. Rehydration: 100 ml/kg 2. Ongoing losses: 30 ml/kg Reassess progress.	NPM for six hours. Then feed as above.

Hypovolaemia: NB: May in fulminant cases not have signs of clinical dehydration!

Over 10% dehydrated Compensated shock, LOC normal, BP diastolic >60 mmHg, peripheral pulses palpable **(Severe)**	1. Ringers lactate or normal saline (N/S) by IV 2. ½ DD by IV 3. ½ DD by IV	1. Resuscitation: 10 ml/kg IV fast (Repeat if needed) 2. Rehydration: 100 ml/kg 3. Ongoing losses: 30 ml/kg Reassess two-hourly till stable.	NPM Feed after 6–12 hours Breast-/bottle feeds: Pelargon®
Over 10% dehydrated Uncompensated shock. Decreased LOC, BP diastolic <60 mmHg, peripheral pulses not palpable **(Very severe)**	1. Ringers Lactate or N/S by IV. NB. Intraosseous if cannot give IV 2. ½ DD 3. ½ DD	1. Resuscitation 20 ml/kg IV fast. Reassess BP / pulses. (Repeat 10 ml/kg IV fast if needed) 2. Rehydration: 100 ml/kg 3. Ongoing losses: 30 ml/kg Reassess two-hourly till stable.	NPM Feed after 6–12 hours as above.

Note: Maintenance fluids – see Table 8.2 on page 168.

In addition to the fluids given on the previous page: Maintenance fluid is given IV or orally as $^1/_2$ DD, ORS, breast or bottle milk (Pelargon®).

Table 8.2 Maintenance volumes per 24 hours

Weight	Volume/24 hours
1–10 kg	100 ml/kg
11–20 kg	1 000 ml plus 50 ml/kg for each kg over 10 kg
21–60 kg	1 500 ml plus 20 ml/kg for each kg over 20 kg

Severe diarrhoea
- Dehydration present with or without vomiting.
- Requires an intragastric drip or IV fluids for rehydration (see Fluid therapy in Table 8.1).

Specific therapy
The role of antibiotics and chemotherapeutic agents remains controversial. They are of no value in the majority of cases and of limited value even in bacterial diarrhoea. However, antibiotics must be used in malnourished, very young (under one month), and potentially septic patients. They should provide cover against both Gram-positive and Gram-negative organisms; amoxycillin (e.g. Amoxil®), and co-trimoxazole (e.g. Septran® and Bactrim®) are suitable preparations. Amoebiasis and giardiasis both respond well to metronidazole (Flagyl®). Other parenteral infections are treated on their own merits.

In lactose intolerance, give a lactose-free milk substitute, for example soya milk that has sucrose as its sugar.

Non-specific anti-diarrhoeal agents, such as kaolin, codeine phosphate, diphenoxylate hydrochloride (Lomotil®) or loperamide hydrochloride (Imodium®) are not recommended for children. They have side effects and often give a false sense of security, as stool numbers may decrease, but fluid loss may remain unchanged with intraluminal bowel stasis.

Fluid therapy
Purpose
Fluid therapy is aimed at the restoration and maintenance of normal water and electrolyte balance. It is of particular importance in paediatric

practice, as infants and children have a high water and electrolyte turnover, and emergency situations occur rapidly.

The best treatment is to give additional oral electrolyte solution before the infant becomes clinically dehydrated.

Methods of fluid therapy

- Oral feeds.
- Intragastric / nasogastric drip.
- Intravenous infusion.
- Intraosseous.

The same general principals apply, whichever route is used and are strongly recommended.

- Intragastric / nasogastric rehydration is commonly and extensively used.
- Intravenous therapy is used in:
  - Acute situations: Treatment of severe dehydration or shock (hypovolaemia).
  - Subacute states: Where oral feeding is inadvisable or impractical, for example severe respiratory disease or protracted vomiting.
  - Chronic states: Where maintenance of hydration and nutrition is impossible by the normal route, for example intractable diarrhoea, post-intestinal surgery.

Fluid requirements consist of:

- Maintenance fluid necessary for maintaining hydration and normal ongoing losses.
- Replacement fluid necessary for restoring hydration to normal, that is:
  - Replacing losses that have already occurred.
  - Ongoing diarrhoeal losses: 30 ml/kg.

Maintenance requirements

Fundamental considerations: The normal ongoing losses that are usually replaced by dietary water and electrolytes are from three major sources:

1. **Insensible water loss:** Mainly from skin and lungs.
2. **Renal loss as urine:** 15–25 ml/kg/24 hours (1 ml/kg/hr).
3. **Gastrointestinal loss:** Under normal circumstances, loss of water from the gastrointestinal tract is small, and in a child may be as low as 5 ml/kg/day. In cases of diarrhoea, however, these losses may be very large indeed; up to 300 ml/kg/day.

Maintenance fluid requirements for intragastric and intravenous therapy (These volumes do not apply to normal oral infant feeds which are 150 ml/kg/day)

The total volume of fluid per day is given using infusion bottles containing small volumes (200 ml), to avoid the danger of inadvertently giving a large amount of intravenous fluid rapidly.

The maintenance requirements given in the table serve as a guide only. Losses from diarrhoea, nasogastric drainage, ileostomy, fistulae, etc. should be measured if possible, and replaced as they occur. Fluid schedules may have to be revised several times daily as the situation changes.

Table 8.3 Maintenance requirements for intragastric and intravenous therapy

	Age	Volume – ml/kg/day
Neonates	1 day	60
	2 days	75
	3 days	100
	4 days	125
	5 days and older	150
	Weight	**Volume/24 hours**
Infants	1–10 kg	100 ml/kg
	11–20 kg	1 000 ml plus 50 ml/kg for each kg over 10 kg
	21–60 kg	1 500 ml plus 20 ml/kg for each kg over 20 kg

Replacement requirements
Fundamental considerations

The signs and symptoms of dehydration are directly proportional to the amount of fluid lost. This is seen as a percentage reduction in body weight. The signs and symptoms are the same at all ages, as the proportion of an individual's body that consists of water changes only slightly over a lifetime. The initial effects of dehydration are haemodynamic rather than metabolic.

The best and most objective method of assessing dehydration is using short-term weight changes. Previous weights are not always available and the amount of replacement fluid then has to be assessed using clinical signs (see Dehydration, p. 162).

Replacement fluids – amount
Aim at complete correction of dehydration in the well-nourished child within 24 hours, and in the malnourished, small or chronically ill child, within 48 hours. Replacement fluids together with the calculated maintenance fluid are given at a steady rate over 24 hours. Preferably err on the side of correcting too slowly, but remember that constant reassessment is necessary, as one must keep ahead of continuing losses.

Replacement amounts are calculated on the estimated percentage of dehydration and body weight, for example 10% of 5 kg = 500 ml.
5%   dehydration = 50 ml/kg
10% dehydration = 100 ml/kg fluid lost (deficit)

Never calculate replacements on more than 10% dehydration. This should avoid the possibility of fluid overload.

Once you have decided how much fluid to give (i.e. maintenance volume for age plus replacement volume based on % dehydration), you must then decide what fluid, at what speed, and by which route.

Specific considerations
• **Shock (hypovolaemia)**
This is a medical emergency, with the need to re-establish the circulating blood volume as rapidly as possible. If IV not possible, see Intraosseous Infusion, p. 359. An isotonic electrolyte solution should be used. Ringers lactate is the fluid of choice but the following can be used:
  ○ Normal Saline.
  ○ Haemaccel®.
  ○ Plasma or Stabilised Human Serum (SHS).
  ○ Plasmalyte B.
  ○ Blood (if indicated).

Volumes: Initially, 10–20 ml/kg of one of the above is given rapidly intravenously and 2 mmol/kg (2 ml/kg) 8% sodium bicarbonate is given simultaneously as a slow IV bolus. The clinical state is then reassessed. If response is inadequate, a further 10 ml/kg fluid may be given rapidly. If shock still persists, it is advisable to monitor further fluid administration with a central venous pressure line (normal CVP = 5–10 cms/water). If CVP is normal and shock continues, IV Dopamine or equivalent is indicated to improve cardiac output.

Once shock has been corrected, or if not initially present, proceed as follows:

• Dehydration

Half-strength Darrows in 5% dextrose solution has been found to be effective in correcting dehydration in most situations. It is contraindicated in anuria because of its potassium content. It is also contraindicated in dehydration due to vomiting, where there is frequently an associated alkalosis, because of its lactate (alkali) content. (In pyloric stenosis, the rehydration fluid of choice is half-strength normal saline.) If there has been prolonged diarrhoea with resultant potassium depletion, it will be necessary to add supplementary potassium chloride orally (0,5 g eight-hourly).

Route of administration: This can be either oral, *via* an intra-gastric drip or intravenously.

Acidosis

If severe (pH less than 7,1), this requires correction with 8% sodium bicarbonate intravenously.

Amount: 2 ml/kg of child's weight (no laboratory facilities), or if Astrup / Blood gas is available, weight in kg × 0,3 × base excess = ml of 8% sodium bicarbonate required.

Give half the calculated amount as a slow IV bolus and reassess again later. Continue rehydrating the patient. The most common cause of persistent acidosis is inadequate rehydration.

If acidosis persists or recurs despite adequate fluid replacement, refer for assessment of renal function.

Hypernatraemia

Suspect hypernatraemia in any child who is very jittery, has convulsions, or has a 'brawny' feel to skin.

Hypernatraemia (serum Na greater than 150 mmol/l) presents a difficult therapeutic problem. Electrolyte transfer is slower than water transfer, and rapidly giving an IV hypotonic electrolyte solution may result in brain swelling and convulsions. Half-strength Darrows in 5% dextrose solution is effective therapy if the replacement and maintenance volumes are given slowly and evenly over 48 hours. A problem arises if there is accompanying shock, as this must be corrected rapidly. In such situations, Ringers lactate is the optimal solution for restoring adequate circulation. If unavailable, all isotonic fluids such as Haemaccel®, plasma or SHS, may be used. Once circulation is restored, further replacement and maintenance can be achieved with half-strength Darrows in 5% dextrose as above. Try to correct acidosis with rehydration only as additional sodium bicarbonate may worsen the hypernatraemia. Urine output must be established and maintained. Put on a urine bag in these cases.

Preventable causes
- Incorrect reconstitution of powdered milk (too strong).
- Giving of too strong home-made oral salt solutions for rehydration therapy ('salt' poisoning).
- Underestimating dehydration in fat infants.

Hypokalaemia
This is more likely to occur in malnourished children. It may be extremely dangerous and can cause cardiac arrest. The older child may present with hypotonia and poor head control. The younger infant may have an ileus; or the condition may only be detected by laboratory and ECG findings. All malnourished children and any child with prolonged diarrhoea must receive additional potassium as potassium chloride by mouth for two or three days.

Dosage of potassium chloride
- If younger than six months: 0,25 g eight-hourly.
- If older than six months: 0,5 g eight-hourly.

Other factors in fluid therapy
Nutrition
Any child on conventional IV therapy is being starved. There is no fat or protein intake and energy requirements are not being met. Plasma 10 ml/kg/day will help to maintain plasma protein, but this does not meet daily protein requirements. A 10% dextrose solution may be used to supply additional calories and prevent hypoglycaemia (particularly in the first few days after birth), but this does not cover all the energy needs.

Intravenous therapy should therefore be kept as brief as possible. If it has to be prolonged, then total intravenous nutrition using amino acid solutions, intravenous fat, and carbohydrate becomes necessary. This technique should only be carried out by experienced personnel.

Vitamins and trace elements
It is necessary to add vitamins if IV therapy is prolonged for more than

three days, in which case the normal requirements are given using an intravenous vitamin preparation (expensive). Trace element requirements can be met by giving plasma at weekly intervals.

Blood transfusion

Never exceed 20 ml of blood/kg body weight unless the patient is actively bleeding, or has a history of major recent blood loss. Anaemia alone is not an indication for blood transfusion. The cause should be investigated prior to the method of treatment being planned. If anaemic and in cardiac failure, packed cells with Lasix® cover should be given.

Fluids in common use

Table 8.4 Fluids in common use

	Sodium	Potassium	Chloride	Lactate
	(mmol per litre)			
½ DD (5% dextrose)	61	17	51	27
Normal saline (0,9%)	154	–	154	–
½ normal saline (0,45%)	77	–	77	–
Haemaccel®	154	5,1	154	–
Ringers lactate	131	5	112	29

Plasma has approximately the same electrolyte content as serum, but the potassium may be much higher.

5% D/W (5 g carbohydrate/100 ml) = 20 kcal/100 ml (1 g carbohydrate = 4 kcals) while 10% D/W = 40 kcal/100 ml. Therefore, at 120 ml/kg/day of 5% dextrose the patient is getting ± 50 kcal/kg/day.

There are no short cuts or rules of the thumb for intelligent fluid therapy. Consideration of the whole problem in each individual patient is essential. Constant reassessment of the child, particularly by clinical examination but also by serum electrolytes and acid-base determinations if necessary, is the key to successful fluid therapy.

Normal caloric requirement is 110 kcals/kg/day. Patient is therefore being starved even if on 10% IV dextrose water.

Rectal prolapse

This commonly occurs in malnourished children with constipation, children with large bulky stools as in malabsorption syndromes (cystic fibrosis), or associated with whooping cough. The prolapsed rectum becomes very oedematous if not replaced reasonably soon. Replace with gentle pressure, and then strap buttocks together with Elastoplast®. Strapping is not always successful. Improve the child's nutrition and also any other underlying factors. If prolapse occurs repeatedly, refer to hospital as surgical fixation may be necessary.

Vomiting

Vomiting is a common symptom throughout childhood and may be associated with a wide variety of diseases of all degrees of severity. Many causes are trivial, but vomiting may indicate serious disease and should never be taken lightly. If vomiting is protracted or severe, the possibility of a serious associated disease must be considered. Vomiting is a symptom, not a diagnosis.

In investigating the cause of vomiting, a careful history and physical examination are essential. Pay special attention to the following:

- Frequency of vomiting.
- Quantity of vomits.
- Contents of vomitus: Food, bile, blood or faecal.
- Character of vomiting: Forcible, with wind, or effortless as in gastro-oesophageal reflux.
- Relation to meals.
- Presence of nausea (as judged by appetite).
- Associated symptoms: Pain, fever, coughing.
- Whether the child is thriving despite the vomiting.

Persistent vomiting of large amounts of food (causing failure to gain weight), vomiting blood or bile, or vomiting associated with abdominal distention and / or constipation must be investigated.

During the neonatal period

Vomiting is a relatively common sign during the neonatal period. In the majority of instances, it is simply regurgitation after a feed and can be prevented by nursing the infant head up and on the abdomen (prone) or left side. When vomiting occurs shortly after birth and is persistent, the possibilities of raised intracranial pressure, oesophageal atresia or intestinal obstruction must be considered.

Common causes

- Swallowing of blood or meconium during birth: These may cause gastritis and the vomitus contains a lot of mucus. It can be treated by washing out the stomach with solution of half normal saline or 2% sodium bicarbonate, followed by breastfeeding.
- Feeding faults:
  - Underfeeding: Hungry and swallows air when fed.
  - Overfeeding: Especially preterm infants.
  - Hole in the teat is too small or too large.

Serious causes

- Infection:
  - Diarrhoeal disease.
  - Septicaemia.
  - Meningitis.
- Raised intracranial pressure:
  - Meningitis.
  - Cerebral irritation: Usually due to difficult delivery with hypoxia, causing haemorrhage or cerebral oedema.
    If associated with convulsions, refer.
- Intestinal obstruction.
- Oesophageal atresia: If this suspected, pass a nasogastric tube and test with litmus paper for acidity. If not acid, nurse head up and refer to hospital, aspirating the pharynx during the journey. Leave the nasogastric tube in place and aspirate often.
- Inborn errors of metabolism: Rare but important.

In early infancy

Common causes

- Possetting, that is, vomiting of small amounts of curdled milk after a feed, is normal.
- Feeding faults:
  - Underfeeding.
  - Overfeeding.
  - Swallowed air (hole in teat too big or too small).
- Gastro-oesophageal reflux.
- Minor infections.

Serious causes
- Acute infective disease; infants may vomit with almost any infectious disease.

Note: Diarrhoeal disease, meningitis, urinary tract infection, throat infection.
- Pyloric stenosis.
- Hiatus hernia.
- Intestinal obstruction.

In late infancy

Common causes
- Acute infective disease, for example meningitis, gastroenteritis.

Less common causes
- Intestinal obstruction, intussusception.
- Poisoning (accidental).
- Food intolerance.
- Rumination (habitual vomiting).

Over two years of age (Childhood)
Mechanical factors and parenteral infections are not so common in this age group.

Common causes
- Acute dietary indiscretion, for example a birthday party.
- Organic disease of the abdomen, for example appendicitis.
- Organic disease of the nervous system, for example meningitis, cerebral tumour.
- Emotional disturbances: Varying from simple excitement to serious psychiatric disturbances of the family dynamics. (Be wary – brain tumours may start like this.)

Less common causes
- Cyclical vomiting / psychogenic.
- Poisoning (food, accidental, suicidal, iatrogenic; child in cardiac failure from digitalis intoxication).
- Metabolic disease, for example diabetes or chronic renal failure.
- Motion sickness (car, air, sea).
- Post-nasal drip.
- Whooping cough.

Examination

Pay particular attention to nutritional status, hydration, ENT, urinary tract, and the abdomen (distension / tenderness, guarding etc.).

Treatment

It is essential that the underlying cause be sought. Phenothiazine derivatives such as Stemetil® are widely used and do relieve vomiting from many causes, but this may obscure serious and correctable causes of vomiting. Metoclopramide (Maxolon® or Primperan®) is a useful medication, but should only be used once organic causes have been excluded.

Any case of vomiting which is bile-stained, persistent, or has caused dehydration must be referred immediately.

Haematology

Normal values

These vary with age.

Table 9.1

Age	Haemoglobin range g/dl
Birth	16–20
3 months	10–12
1 year	10–13
2 years	12–14
4 years	12–14
8–12 years	12–15

The normally high haemoglobin concentration at birth falls steadily to reach a low point at about 3 months. During this period, the bone marrow is relatively inactive, allowing the haemoglobin to fall. Thereafter, it becomes active again and the haemoglobin rises.

Blood cells and their function

Red blood cells

The main role of red cells is to carry oxygen by means of haemoglobin from the lungs to the tissues for the normal functioning of the body. They also carry carbon dioxide from the tissues to the lungs where it is exhaled. This carbon dioxide is a very important by-product of metabolism.

White blood cells

The white cells are responsible for resistance to infection and for removing the products of cellular breakdown in the body. They consist of one group called granulocytes, which are mainly polymorphs.

Their function is to phagocytose and destroy bacteria. In this group, eosinophils are also important in allergic reactions. The other group is the non-granulocytes which consist of macrophages and lymphocytes. Some lymphocytes which live a long time are called memory cells and are important in immunoglobulin production (B-cells) and cellular immunity (T-cells).

Platelets

These are small fragments which are essential in the clotting process. If any vessel is injured, they stick to the injured part and stimulate blood clotting in that area to stop further bleeding. Platelets repair small holes in the capillary walls.

Blood disorders

Anaemia

Definition

A haemoglobin value below the lower limit of the normal range for age indicates anaemia. For full understanding of the type and cause of anaemia, further tests must be done, including chemical and microscopic examination of the blood, and sometimes examination of the bone marrow.

There are four general ways in which children may become anaemic:

1. Shortage of one of the materials needed to make haemoglobin in the bone marrow:
   - Iron.
   - Protein (as in kwashiorkor).
   - Folic acid.
   - Vitamin B_{12} (rare).

2. 'Sick Marrow'
   The bone marrow is inactive, and thus does not make enough red cells, even though all materials are available. The causes are:
   - Chronic disease, for example renal failure or rheumatoid arthritis.
   - Marrow toxins, for example chloramphenicol, cytotoxic drugs.
   - Marrow replaced by malignant cells, for example leukaemia.

3. Excessive breakdown of red cells once they have been made and released into the blood stream, as in the haemolytic anaemias, for example Rhesus and ABO incompatibility, thalassaemia, sickle cell

anaemia, or malaria, where red cells are destroyed by the malaria parasite.

4. Blood loss, especially as nosebleeds, or from gastrointestinal tract.

All anaemias have a cause which must be found. There is no place for accepting a simple descriptive diagnosis of anaemia. The question, 'Why did this child become anaemic?' must always be asked and answered.

Clinical features of anaemia of any cause
- Tiredness.
- Irritability.
- Poor feeding.
- Pale conjunctivae, nail beds, and tongue.
- Palmar pallor (i.e. pale palms).

If anaemia is severe, the child may become breathless due to heart failure.

Iron-deficiency anaemia
Definition
This is a result of insufficient iron being available for the manufacture of haemoglobin by the bone marrow.

Epidemiology
- Worldwide. The most common cause of anaemia in children.
- Common in areas of low socio-economic status, where nutrition is poor and the prevalence of intestinal parasites is high.
- Prevalent between six months and three years.

Iron physiology
Iron in the diet is absorbed from the upper small intestine and stored for later use. These stores consist of:
- Certain blood proteins.
- Special storage cells in the bone marrow.

When a child becomes iron deficient, the iron stored in the above sites is mobilised and used to make red cells. Only when these stores are depleted does the production of haemoglobin fall and the child becomes clinically anaemic. This is why, when treating a child for iron deficiency anaemia, it is necessary to continue the iron therapy for a month or two after the haemoglobin is back to normal in order to refill the iron stores.

Aetiology
There are three main causes.

1. Insufficient iron absorbed from the intestine
This usually means the diet is short of iron. In rare cases, the gastrointestinal tract may be diseased and unable to absorb enough iron (malabsorption). Meat, eggs, green vegetables, and certain fruits are iron-rich, but milk and porridge contain little iron. A toddler on a diet of milk and porridge and very little else soon becomes iron deficient.

2. Iron loss
This is nearly always due to chronic blood loss. The most common causes of blood loss are intestinal parasites (e.g. *Trichuris trichiura*) and gastrointestinal haemorrhage (e.g. from oesophageal varices). Blood loss during menstrual periods in adolescent girls may cause anaemia if the diet contains too little iron.

3. Low iron stores in preterm infants
The normal term infant gets most of his or her stores of iron from the mother during the last four weeks of pregnancy. These are sufficient to last for the first six months of life, by which time the child will be on an iron-containing mixed diet. Preterm infants miss these final four weeks of pregnancy and so are born with inadequate iron stores. They become iron-deficient in the first few months of life if additional iron is not given.

Clinical features
As for anaemia generally, although mild cases are often undetected clinically. Splenomegaly occurs in about 10% of cases.

Management of iron deficiency anaemia
- Check stools for blood (Haematest®).
- Find and treat the cause, for example diet, parasites, etc.
- Ferrous sulphate syrup (20 mg iron/5 ml). Dose 6 mg/kg/day. In general, 5 to 10 ml in three equal doses between meals. Ferrous lactate drops (0,6 ml) twice daily may be used in infants. Stools may go grey or dark brown. Continue for one month after haemoglobin is back to normal.

- Haemoglobin should rise 1 to 2 g/dl per week if the treatment is adequate.
- Advise on diet if necessary.
- Follow-up monthly for six months to ensure that the haemoglobin does not fall again.

Iron supplements for infants:
Full term and particularly preterm infants, whether breast- or bottle-fed, should receive an iron supplement until solid feeds are introduced. Term infants need 0,3 ml Ferrodrops® (1 mg/kg/day), while preterm infants need 0,6 ml Ferrodrops® (2 mg/kg/day) daily from two weeks onwards.

Advice to parents and treatment
- Explain nature and course of condition.
- Advise about the value of green vegetables, liver, eggs, etc. in the diet.
- Prevent iron poisoning by keeping out of reach of children.
- The patient must return in two weeks for haemoglobin check.
- If no increase in haemoglobin after iron treatment for two weeks, refer for more detailed investigation.
- The importance of taking medication for a long period must be stressed.
- Warn that colour of stool may change to grey or even black.

Indications for referral
- No response of haemoglobin to ferrous sulphate after two weeks.
- Purpura.
- Hepatosplenomegaly.
- Haematuria.
- If haemoglobin is below 7,5 g/dl.

Bleeding disorders
These are not very common, but it is essential to recognise them when they occur as they can be extremely dangerous. In many cases, there may be a family history to alert you to the condition in the child. Remember that a toxic and ill child who haemorrhages may have the highly infectious condition of haemorrhagic (Congo) fever.

Special note must be taken of the child who bruises easily (out of proportion to nature or degree of injury), or who bleeds into muscles or into joints. Other signs of a bleeding disorder may be bleeding excessively after a tooth extraction, circumcision, or minor lacerations. All these cases must be referred for further investigation.

Purpura

Purple or dark red skin lesions from bleeding into skin which do not fade on pressure.

If the lesions are very small, they are called petechiae (look like pin pricks). Large lesions are called ecchymoses (bruises).

Aetiology

There are many causes, most of which are serious.

- As the result of damage to capillaries, for example in septicaemias. The infecting organism damages the small blood vessels, causing bleeding. The most important example is meningococcaemia.
- As a result of too few platelets. Reduced numbers occur in conditions such as:
  - Idiopathic thrombocytopenic purpura.
  - Leukaemia.
  - Aplastic anaemia.
  - Drug reactions.

The importance of recognising purpura lies in the fact that it nearly always means a serious disease that needs urgent referral. Meningococcaemia is a true emergency.

Chapter 10

Infectious diseases

General approach to any infectious disease
Clinical features

These are often the means by which a diagnosis is made. The child may first be seen during any of the following clinical stages:
- Incubation period.
- Prodromal period (stage of invasion).
- Stage of advance.
- Complications.

Findings on examination may be general (non-specific), or specific for that infectious disease.

Laboratory tests

These are usually of value in confirming the clinical diagnosis. Tests include direct staining methods, bacterial or viral isolation, and serological tests.

Common aspects and stages of any infectious disease

- Aetiological or causative organism (e.g. bacterial or viral).
- Method of transmission.
- Specific incubation period.
- Specific pathology.
- Special clinical findings during:
  - Prodromal period.
  - Stage of advance.
- Complications.
- Treatment:
  - Prevention.
  - Specific.

o Supportive.
• Period of isolation (infectious period).

Infectious diseases that must be notified to the local health authority

Cholera
Congenital syphilis
Diphtheria
Haemorrhagic fever
Lead poisoning
Leprosy
Malaria
Measles
Meningococcal meningitis (including meningococcaemia)
Poisoning from any agricultural or stock remedy
Poliomyelitis (any case of flaccid paralysis)
Rabies
Rheumatic fever / heart disease
Tetanus
Tuberculosis
Typhoid fever
Viral hepatitis A, B, and other

Skin rashes

These occur in a number of infectious diseases and, depending on when they are seen, may cause difficulty in interpretation. This is especially true in dark-skinned children.

The rashes may be caused by:
• Bacteria or viruses acting directly on capillaries (vasculitis).
• Toxins of bacteria or viruses acting on capillaries: An example is the exotoxin of scarlet fever.
• Mechanical causes, for example from venous congestion due to paroxysms of coughing in whooping cough when small purpuric spots on face may occur.
• Secondary changes in rashes altering their original appearance, for example secondary infection of skin lesions in chicken pox.

Table 10.1 Stages of infectious diseases

	Incubation period	Prodromal period	Isolation period
Short			
Gastroenteritis	1–7 days	Nil	Till diarrhoea stops
Diphtheria	1–7 days	Nil	Till three throat swabs are negative
Influenza	1–7 days	Nil	Till apyrexial and feeling better
Meningococcal	1–7 days	Nil	2 days from start of disease treatment
Scarlet fever	1–7 days	Nil	Till rash fades and desquamation starts
Intermediate			
Measles	7–14 days	3–7 days	5 days from start of rash
Pertussis	7–14 days	Up to 21 days; usually 5–7 days	4–6 weeks or for first 2 days of treatment with erythromycin
Polio	7–14 days	3–36 days	10 days
Tetanus	7–14 days	Nil	Not required
Typhoid	7–14 days	Nil (diagnosis difficult in early stages of disease)	Till 3 consecutive stool cultures are negative

Long			
Chickenpox	14–21 days	0–2 days	Till lesions crusted; usually 5–7 days
Hepatitis A	15–50 days	2–5 days	7 days from onset of jaundice
Hepatitis B	50–180 days	2–5 days	Till no longer jaundiced
Mumps	14–21 days	0–1 days	Till swelling subsides
Rubella	14–21 days	0–2 days	Nil, except from pregnant women for approximately 7 days

The stage of a rash occurring in the mouth is called the enanthema (e.g. as seen in Koplik's spots inside the mouth in early measles). The main skin rash is known as the exanthema and goes through various stages of development, followed by healing.

Immunisation

Schedules

The following is the current schedule recommended by the South African Department of National Health.

Age	**Vaccine**
Birth	TOPV(O), BCG
6 weeks	TOPV(1), DPT(1), HBV(1)HIB(1)
10 weeks	TOPV(2), DPT(2), HBV(2)HIB(2)
14 weeks	TOPV(3), DPT(3), HBV(3)HIB(3)
9 months	Measles(1)
18 months	TOPV(4), DPT(4), Measles(2)
5 years	TOPV(5), DT

Abbreviations

TOPV	Trivalent Oral Polio Vaccine
DPT	Diphtheria, Pertussis, and Tetanus Vaccine
DT	Diphtheria and Tetanus Vaccine (no pertussis)
HBV	Hepatitis B Vaccine
HIB	Haemophilus Influenzae Type B Vaccine
BCG	Bacillus Calmette Guerin (Tuberculosis Vaccine)

If, for some reason, the child should start immunisation after infancy, the following schedule is recommended:

First visit	DPT + trivalent polio + measles
Six weeks later	DPT + trivalent polio + BCG
Six weeks thereafter	DPT + trivalent polio
Twelve months later	DPT + trivalent polio

Pertussis vaccine should not be given after 18 months.

General points about the schedule

If vaccination schedule is interrupted, it can be completed at any time later; it is not necessary to start from the beginning. The efficacy of vaccines is not affected by giving several simultaneously. If in doubt as to whether BCG has been given previously, it may be given at same time as DPT and polio. Live vaccines may be given at the same time without loss of efficiency.

General contraindications to immunisation

- During an acute severe illness.
- If the child has received gamma globulin, plasma or blood transfusion within the previous eight weeks.
- In immunodeficiency disorders. In general this does not include HIV/AIDS.
- If on immunosuppressive medications (these include corticosteroids, cytotoxics, as well as radiotherapy).
- In the presence of any malignant disease process (includes leukaemia).
- If the child has a progressive (i.e. gradually worsening) neurological disorder or history of convulsions, the pertussis part of DPT must not be given.

- If any DPT injection was followed by a convulsion, omit pertussis fraction thereafter.

> **Note:** Minor illnesses such as coughs or colds, or treatment with antibiotics, *are not contraindications to immunisation.*

Recording of immunisation

It is essential to fill out the immunisation section of a child's Road to Health card when immunisation procedures are done. If this is impossible, at least give the parent a form, stating the date and procedure. It is compulsory to inform local authorities about all procedures carried out.

Open vial policy

In South Africa there is a strict policy relating to the use of open vials of vaccine. It is essential that this policy is adhered to, in order to ensure that the infant receives a safe, effective vaccine.

All open vials must have the date and time written on the label when it is opened.

The individual open vaccines must be discarded after a specific period:
- **BCG**: Discard six hours after opening.
- **Measles**: Discard six hours after opening.
- **DPT HIB combined**: Discard seven days after opening.
- **HIB not combined with DPT**: Discard seven days after opening.
- **DPT not combined with HIB**: Discard one month after opening.
- **Tetanus toxoid**: Discard one month after opening.
- **HEP B**: Discard one month after opening.

This rule does not apply to polio vaccine vials. Polio has its own vaccine vial monitor on each vial (as well as expiry date). As soon as the inner square matches the outer, the polio vaccine must not be used.

All vaccines used in mobile clinics must be discarded at the end of the session.

General principles: Handling and storage of live vaccines (BCG, measles and polio, MMR)

- Store at 2–8 °C (only polio vaccine may be frozen).
- Avoid direct sunlight as it kills the organisms.
- Do not clean vials with alcohol, ether or spirits, as these agents may kill the organisms.

Vaccines

BCG vaccine

Given at birth. If missed at birth, it can be given until 12 months of age. The vaccine is a freeze-dried, live attenuated preparation of the bacillus Calmette Guerin. It should be stored in a refrigerator at 2–8 °C. It should not be frozen and must be kept out of direct sunlight. The diluent should be stored in a cool place. The vaccine is reconstituted with diluent. The vial should not be cleaned with alcohol, as it may kill the vaccine. The vaccine will last for eight hours in a refrigerator after reconstitution if kept in the dark. (See manufacturer's instructions, as conditions are different for different makes.)

Method of administration

In South Africa the route of BCG administration changed from percutaneous to intradermal in 2001.
- Clean the right upper arm with soap and water.
- Administer 0,05 ml of the reconstituted BCG vaccine intradermally over the deltoid.
- Do not apply waterproof dressing after administration as this can delay healing.

Contraindications

As for general immunisation (see p. 189).
- Delay for two months after infection with measles.
- In the presence of burns.
- Patient with symptomatic AIDS.

Note: It may be given to malnourished children and preterm babies (when discharged from hospital).

Side effects

In 1–2% of infants, ulceration at the site of immunisation and local lymphadenitis may occur. This is more common in children with HIV.

DPT *vaccine*

This contains:

- Diphtheria toxoid
- Tetanus toxoid   Absorbed on aluminium
- Extract of killed   phosphate gel.
  Pertussis bacteria

Storage

- In refrigerator or cold box at 2–8 °C. It is important not to freeze, as this causes irreversible clumping of gel and leads to irregular dosage and cyst formation.
- Avoid direct sunlight.

Method of administration

- The normal vial holds 10 ml and is ready for use.
- Shake the vial to disperse colloids before withdrawing each dose to prevent sterile abscess formation.
- Use a fresh syringe and a new 23 gauge needle for each child.
- Swab clean.

Dosage

0,5 ml IM given into the deltoid or quadriceps muscle.

Contraindications

As for general immunisation (see p. 189).

Previous severe reaction to DPT injection, including anaphylaxis, collapse, persistent screaming, a fever over 40 °C, convulsions within three days, encephalopathy within seven days. In these cases, drop the pertussis fraction for subsequent injections.

Side effects

- Local: Mild induration and tenderness at injection site.
- Systemic reaction: Low grade fever is fairly common.
- More serious side effects such as convulsions and encephalitis are very rare and are most probably due to the pertussis element.

Td *vaccine*

This is used for children over ten years as a booster, or for primary immunisation if the schedule has not already begun. The vaccine contains a reduced dose of both diphtheria toxoid and absorbed tetanus toxoid on aluminium phosphate gel. It is not available in South Africa presently.

Dosage
0,5 ml IM into the deltoid (it is important to shake the vial first).

Poliomyelitis vaccine (Sabin)
The trivalent polio vaccine is used. It contains a mixture of Types 1, 2, and 3 of the poliomyelitis virus strain.

Storage
Long-term
Kept in the deep freeze at –20 °C, where it lasts for up to two years.

Short-term
Main compartment of a refrigerator (2–8 °C). Once the vaccine has thawed, it must not be frozen as this kills the virus. It is convenient to keep the vial in a refrigerator or cool bag when in use.

Note: Direct sunlight kills the virus.

Method of administration
Shake bottle; put two drops directly into the mouth from the plastic dropper bottle.

Contraindications
As for general immunisation (see p. 189)

Diarrhoea may lead to poor colonisation of bowel by the polio vaccine virus, and is a relative contraindication. However, in a high-risk situation, it is advised that the vaccine should be given, and arrangements be made for an extra dose to be given after the diarrhoea has stopped.

Measles vaccine
The present vaccine is a freeze-dried attenuated measles virus (Schwarz strain), which is reconstituted with a special diluent supplied with the vaccine.

Schedule

- Routinely given at nine and 18 months.
- In high-risk areas and in epidemics, it should be given at six months and then again at nine and 18 months. In high-risk areas, it is important to give the vaccine to any child over the age of five months if being admitted to a hospital ward, attending a clinic, or a hospital outpatients department. These places are the greatest sources of cross-infection with measles. The mechanism to carry this out reliably must be built into the running of health care facilities.

Storage

It is important to protect the vaccine from heat and light which kill the virus. Store between 2–8 °C in a refrigerator or a cold box. The diluent should be stored in the same way.

Method of administration

- Reconstitute vaccine with diluent (use 5 ml for the 10-dose vial). Do not use spirits or ether to clean top of vial, as this may kill the virus.
- Reconstituted vaccine will usually last for six hours if kept cool and out of direct sunshine.
- Use a fresh syringe and needle for each patient.
- Draw up a dose per child and administer it immediately. Do not draw up a dose long before administering it.

Dosage

0,5 ml IM into lateral aspect of the thigh.

Contraindications

As for general immunisation (see p. 189).

- A previous anaphylactic reaction to egg products (very rare). Lesser reactions to egg products do not constitute a contraindication.

Note: Mild febrile illnesses such as a coryza, bronchitis, diarrhoea, or otitis media are not contraindications.

Side effects

Fever in 10–20% of cases occurring some five to ten days after vaccine is given. A faint rash is much less common. CNS manifestations are rare, but may occur within 30 days; encephalopathy occurs at a rate of about one case per million doses. SSPE occurs very rarely and begins years later.

Other vaccines available

- **Measles, mumps, rubella (MMR)**: Can be given at 15 months instead of measles alone, and provides life-long protection. This is not given routinely in state clinics but can be purchased and given by GPs.
- **Rubella**: All pubertal girls who have not had MMR should ideally be immunised. This involves a single dose.
- **Influenza**: This is used in epidemic situations, or for protection of patients with chronic severe respiratory or cardiac conditions.
- **Hepatitis B**: Is part of routine schedule and is given with DPT at six, ten, and 14 weeks intramuscularly.
- **Haemophilus influenza B (HiB) vaccine**: This newly available vaccine protects the young infant from serious Haemophilus B infection, particularly meningitis, epiglottitis, and pneumonia in the first two years of life.
  It is given as three doses at the same time as the first three DPT and HEP B doses (six, ten, and 14 weeks). HiB is available alone or combined with DPT.
- **Pneumococcal vaccine** to prevent pneumonia.

Specific infectious diseases

AIDS
See Chapter 11.

Chickenpox (Varicella)
Definition
A mild but highly infectious disease characterised by a rash which appears mostly on the trunk and face. The lesions appear in successive crops, starting as papules and passing through stages of vesicles, pustules, and crusts.

Aetiology
Chickenpox is caused by the varicella-zoster virus, and is primarily an infection of the upper respiratory tract. It is mainly a disease of childhood. Transmission is by air (droplet spread), hands or clothing. It is highly infectious.

Incubation period
Long (from 14–21 days).

Isolation period

Patients are non-infective when the last crop of pustules are scabbed, but schools often do not accept cases back before the last scabs are shed.

Clinical course and findings

The clinical manifestations of chickenpox range from very mild to extremely severe. Generally very young infants and children with immune compromise, such as HIV infection, suffer more severely.

The prodromal phase

This is marked by pyrexia, malaise, headaches, pains in the limbs, nausea, and vomiting. It lasts for 24 hours before the rash appears. In young children it is often absent, and the disease starts with the appearance of the rash.

Stage of advance

The rash starts with macules which soon become papular. Within a few hours, the papules become superficial vesicles (which break easily), then form pustules, and finally become scabs over the next two to four days. The lesions appear first on the back, then the chest, abdomen, face, and scalp. The distal extremities are spared except in severe cases. Lesions may also occur in the mouth. Crops of lesions at different stages of development are typical of chickenpox. Pitting and scarring of the skin results from scratching and secondary infection. If this can be prevented, scarring will not occur.

Complications

These are rare, but the following may occur:
- Impetigo and cellulitis due to secondary streptococcal or staphylococcal infections.
- Primary chickenpox pneumonia.
- Encephalomyelitis may develop four to six days after appearance of the rash; there is a 10% mortality, but survivors usually recover completely.
- Children on corticosteroid and immunosuppressive therapy, for example children with leukaemia, severe malnutrition or HIV disease, may get a fulminating disseminated type of chickenpox with haemorrhagic lesions in the skin and viscera, as well as severe pneumonia which may be fatal.

Diagnosis
This is made on the typical clinical picture. Viral culture and antibody titres can be done in exceptional cases.

Treatment
Supportive:
- Analgesics if necessary.
- Prevent scratching by covering hands in small children. Soothe itching with cool soda bicarbonate baths, calamine lotion or baby powder. If itching is severe, an anti-pruritic such as Vallergan® or Phenergan® syrup may be necessary.
- If secondary infection occurs, treat with an appropriate antibiotic such as penicillin. A local antiseptic such as Cetavlon® or Hibitane® cream can be applied directly to the skin lesions.
- If painful mouth lesions occur, give a fluid diet for a few days.

Specific:
Treatment with acyclovir (Zovirax®) is indicated in encephalitis, pneumonitis, severe or haemorrhagic chickenpox, and in immunocompromised patients including those with HIV/AIDS.

Prevention
- No preventive measures are necessary in healthy children.
- A live attenuated chicken pox virus vaccine is now available but is not given routinely in state clinics; it is reserved for children with malignancy.
- In immunecompromised children, for example those on steroid or immunosuppresive therapy, or severely malnourished children, zoster immune globulin (ZIG) can be given within 72 hours to prevent the disease after contact with an infected person. Ordinary pooled immunoglobulin is not effective in preventing the disease.

Herpes zoster (Shingles)
This is a local manifestation of a reactivated infection with the chicken pox virus. Vesicles are limited to the skin areas supplied by the sensory nerves of a single or associated group of segments of the spinal cord. Lesions appear in crops along the nerve pathways. Chickenpox can occur after exposure to a case of herpes zoster, but not vice versa. Severe pain and paraesthesia are uncommon in children; it occurs mostly in older persons.

Treatment is supportive, with analgesics and local calamine.

Cholera

Definition

Cholera is an acute intestinal disease characterised by the sudden onset of profuse watery stools, vomiting, rapid dehydration, acidosis, and circulatory collapse. Mortality in untreated cases may exceed 50%. Mild cases with diarrhoea do occur, especially in children. It resembles acute infantile gastroenteritis in the profuse and watery nature of the diarrhoea but cholera is not restricted to infants.

Aetiology

Vibrio cholerae is the causative organism. Cholera is still endemic in some areas, for example Southeast Asia. Sporadic epidemics occur from time to time in parts of South Africa. Even in severe epidemics, clinical manifestation rarely exceeds 2% of the population, although subclinical infection rates are much higher.

Transmission

It occurs through ingestion of contaminated water and food. Contamination may be by faeces or vomitus, soiled hands or flies. Poor sanitation and hygiene play an important role in the spread of the disease.

Incubation period

Short (from a few hours to five days, usually two or three days).

Isolation period

This is unknown, but probably for the duration of the stool-positive carrier state which usually lasts for a few days after recovery.

Clinical course and findings

- Prodromal phase: None.
- Stage of advance consists of an acute onset of diarrhoea and vomiting.
- Complications are dehydration, acidosis, and electrolyte disturbances, followed by death in some untreated cases.

Diagnosis

- Clinical: The clinical picture is non-specific.
- Laboratory: Cholera organisms may be cultured from faeces or vomitus or by demonstrating a significant rise in titre of antibodies in acute and convalescent sera.

Treatment
- Supportive treatment is essential and lifesaving and is the mainstay of management. Prompt intravenous therapy of electrolyte solutions (see Fluid therapy, p. 168) to correct dehydration, acidosis, and electrolyte disturbances can lower the mortality to less than 1%.
- Ciprofloxacin or ofloxacin are effective first-line choices for antibiotics. Doxycycline is an appropriate first-line choice in older children and adolescents.

Prevention
- Sanitary disposal of human faeces.
- Protection, purification, and boiling of water.
- Personal hygiene, for example washing of hands before eating and after defecation.
- Chemoprophylaxis of household contacts will reduce the number of cases. Doxycycline is used in two daily doses for two days (per dose 500 mg for adults, 125 mg for children 3 to 13 years, and 50 mg for children under 3).
- Active immunisation of persons at special risk can be carried out but it gives only partial immunity for approximately six months.

Note: Cholera is a notifiable disease.

Diarrhoeal disease
See Gastrointestinal system, p. 161.

Diphtheria
Definition
Diphtheria is an acute infectious disease usually characterised by a local lesion consisting of a membrane in the pharynx or upper respiratory tract. The constitutional symptoms are due to circulating exotoxin which affects nerve tissue and heart muscle.

Aetiology
The disease is caused by the bacteria *Corynebacterium diphtheriae*.

Transmission
Transmission is from person to person, through direct contact or soiled articles.

Incubation period
Short (from one to seven days; usually two to four days).

Isolation period
Patients should be isolated until three consecutive throat swabs, taken 24 hours apart after stopping treatment, are negative.

Clinical course and findings
Prodromal phase: None. Onset usually insidious.

Stage of advance: A white, grey or blackish membrane usually develops within 24 hours. It may be:
- In the nose, where it is often associated with a blood-stained discharge.
- In the throat, where it may spread from the tonsils on to the fauces with marked redness and oedema. Removal of the membrane causes bleeding. Neck glands may be markedly enlarged, causing a 'bull-neck' appearance.
- In the larynx and trachea causing stridor.
- Non-respiratory, for example ear, conjunctiva, skin or genitalia.

Generally, the larger the membrane, the greater the area for toxin absorption, and the more severe the disease.

Complications:
- Death may occur from:
  - Toxaemia towards the end of the first week.
  - Cardiac failure from toxic myocarditis, usually during the second week of the illness.
  - Respiratory failure from peripheral neuritis affecting the vagus nerve, from the third to seventh week (usually the sixth week).
- Myocarditis may present with pallor, small rapid pulse, cardiac failure or peripheral circulatory collapse. Bradycardia or irregular pulse is a serious sign, and indicates damage to cardiac muscle and conductive tissues.
- Paralysis tends to appear in the following order:
  - The palate from the second to third week: This gives a nasal quality to speech and causes regurgitation of fluids.
  - The eyes from the fourth to fifth week: This gives blurred vision due to lack of accommodation. The external muscles are seldom involved.
  - The heart, larynx, and diaphragm with respiratory paralysis from the sixth to seventh weeks.

o Peripheral neuritis with weakness or paralysis of the limbs from the seventh week onwards.

The sensory system is not involved. There is a total absence of permanent damage if death does not occur.

Diagnosis

- Diagnosis is made on the clinical appearance of membrane, oedema, cervical nodes, and a high degree of suspicion. Previous immunisation modifies the clinical picture. Patient may appear surprisingly well.
- Culture of the organism is essential for a firm diagnosis. Direct smear and staining may yield an immediate positive result. Best results are obtained when part of the membrane can be obtained for culture. A negative culture does not exclude the diagnosis. The clinical picture is more important.

Differential diagnosis

Firstly from other diseases which may produce a membrane in the throat:

- Streptococcal throat infection or retropharyngeal or peritonsillar abscess.
- Viral infections, for example herpetic stomatitis or Vincent's angina.
- Fungal infections, for example moniliasis.
- Glandular fever (infective mononucleosis).
- Agranulocytosis or leukaemia.

As it may present with stridor, be particularly suspicious in all cases of laryngotracheobronchitis.

Treatment

Specific:

- Diphtheria antitoxin should be given as early as possible, as circulating toxin becomes fixed in the tissues where antitoxin cannot neutralise it. Dosage varies according to the severity of the infection. Antitoxin may cause severe reactions in individuals sensitised to horse serum products.
- Penicillin therapy should be started early as well. If allergic to penicillin, erythromycin can be given.
- Refer all cases to hospital.

Supportive:

- Absolute bed rest is essential for at least two to three weeks to prevent death from myocarditis.

- Cardiac failure should be treated in the usual way.
- Respiratory failure may require positive pressure ventilation.

Prevention
Diphtheria can be effectively prevented by immunisation during infancy.

Note: Diphtheria is a notifiable disease.

Erythema infectiosum (Slapped cheek disease)
Definition
A common, acute viral disease presenting with a fever and rash.

Aetiology
Parvovirus B 19.

Incubation period
Between one and four weeks.

Isolation period
None, except from pregnant women.

Clinical presentation
- Usually affects young children. Often asymptomatic.
- Fever is either mild or absent.
- Starts with an erythematous rash on face (slapped cheek appearance), which is followed by a macular erythematous rash on the trunk.
- The rash fades from the centre leaving a characteristic 'lacy' appearance to the fading rash.
- The rash is often mildly itchy.
- Resolves spontaneously in a few days.

Complications
- Causes arthritis in rare cases.
- During pregnancy, the virus may infect the fetus, causing severe anaemia, heat failure, and death.
- May cause severe anaemia in infants with chronic haemolytic anaemia, for example thalassaemia.

Treatment
Supportive, with antipyretics.

Food poisoning

Staphylococcal food poisoning

Definition

Staphylococcal food poisoning is characterised by acute nausea, vomiting, cramps, and diarrhoea. Prostration, subnormal temperature, and shock may occur. This is the result of a toxin produced by some strains of the bacteria *Staphylococcus aureus*. It typically occurs in small outbreaks associated with functions such as weddings, where infected food is eaten.

Aetiology

The staphylococci multiply in the food and produce the poisonous enterotoxins which are stable at boiling temperature.

Transmission

By ingestion of food products contaminated by staphylococci from infected hands, nasal secretions, etc.

Incubation period

This is characteristically very short – one to six hours.

Isolation period

None.

Clinical course and findings

- Prodromal stage: None.
- Stage of advance: As above.
- Complications: Dehydration and shock. Death rarely occurs.

Diagnosis

- This is suggested when the typical features occur in a group of people ingesting the same food. Individual cases are seldom recognised as food poisoning.
- Laboratory diagnosis is by culture of faeces, vomitus, and all foodstuffs involved.

Treatment

- Supportive treatment is the most urgent. Give intravenous fluids to correct dehydration and electrolyte disturbances. Treat shock if it occurs.

- Specific: Antibiotics against staphylococci.

Prevention

- Prompt refrigeration of food, for example sliced meats, custards, and cream fillings to avoid multiplication of staphylococci.
- People with purulent skin infections should not be allowed to handle foodstuffs. Food handlers with respiratory infections should wear face masks.
- Meticulous attention to cleanliness in all food handlers.

Clostridium food poisoning

Definition

A disorder characterised by sudden onset of abdominal colic followed by diarrhoea usually accompanied by nausea and vomiting. As with staphylococcal food poisoning, it tends to occur in outbreaks related to consumption of infected food or water.

Aetiology

Infection with *Clostridium perfringens (welchii)*. The symptoms are due both to the infecting organism itself as well as the release of a toxin.

Transmission

This is *via* the ingestion of food, usually meat, contaminated by faeces or soil.

Incubation period

Short (from 12–24 hours).

Isolation period

Unknown.

Clinical course and findings

- Prodromal: None.
- Stage of advance: Sudden onset of abdominal colic followed by diarrhoea. It is usually a mild disease of duration, less than one day. It is rarely fatal in healthy persons.
- Complications: Dehydration and loss of electrolytes.

Diagnosis

- Usually on the basis of the typical clinical picture in a group of people ingesting the same food.

- Laboratory examination and anaerobic culture of food and stools are essential for a definitive diagnosis.

Treatment
- Supportive: Intravenous fluids and electrolytes as required.
- Specific: Usually self-limiting and does not require antibiotics.

Prevention
As for Staphylococcal food poisoning.

Viral hepatitis

The term viral hepatitis usually refers to one of two conditions:
- Hepatitis A (Infectious hepatitis).
- Hepatitis B (Serum hepatitis).

Other forms of hepatitis also occur but are much less common.

Table 10.2 Hepatitis A and B

	Hepatitis A	**Hepatitis B**
Incubation	15–50 days, usually about 1 month	50–180 days
Age	Usually children	Any age
Route of infection	Usually oral	Either oral or parenteral
Hepatitis B surface Ag (HBsAG)	Negative	Positive

Individuals working in children's hospitals are particularly likely to get hepatitis A, while individuals working in renal dialysis units are particularly liable to hepatitis B.

Pathology

Hepatitis A and B both consist of acute inflammation of the whole liver. There may be changes in other organs, for example splenomegaly due to cellular proliferation and venous congestion.

Clinical features

This is a common infection in children, and often occurs in a very mild degree with no symptoms at all and no jaundice. Other cases are more severe with an illness with obvious jaundice. In very few cases there is total liver failure with a high mortality.

In clinically significant cases the clinical picture is as follows:
- **First or pre-icteric phase:** This starts with loss of appetite, nausea, and vomiting, sometimes with a dull ache under the ribs on the right side. This stage may last for up to ten days, but may be completely absent, the child merely feeling ill with headache and some fever.
- **Second or icteric phase:** The urine becomes dark and the stools pale. Jaundice appears and is seen in the 'whites' of the eyes. The liver enlarges and is tender, and the spleen may be enlarged and palpable. By this time the fever, nausea, and loss of appetite usually improve.
- **Third or convalescent phase:** The urine becomes lighter, the stools darker, and jaundice fades. Appetite improves and the child feels well again. The post-hepatitis fatigue and depression of adults are seldom seen in children.

Diagnosis
Mild cases:
- Diagnosed clinically, blood tests unnecessary.
- Bile and urobilinogen in the urine in pre-icteric phase.
- Absent urobilinogen when jaundiced.

More severe cases:
Course is prolonged (over four weeks) or complications occur. Indications for referral to hospital:
- Excess vomiting.
- Signs of liver failure:
  ○ Drowsiness.
  ○ Tremor.
  ○ Ataxia (unsteady gait).
- Failure of jaundice to clear after four weeks.
- Signs of chronic liver disease:
  ○ Very hard liver with or without splenomegaly.
  ○ Ascites.
  ○ Clubbing.
  ○ Oedema.

Investigations
- **Serum bilirubin**: Usually raised (both components).
- **Serum transaminases**: Raised in the illness only.

- **Alkaline phosphatase**: Slightly raised.
- **Serum protein**: This is usually normal, but if disease is prolonged, there may be a fall in albumin and a rise in globulin.
- **Prothrombin time**: Prolonged in severe cases.
- **Blood glucose**: Decreased in severe cases.
- **Hepatitis-related antigens and antibodies**.

Treatment of acute hepatitis

- There is no specific treatment available, so treatment is mainly supportive and symptomatic.
- Give plenty of liquids and small nutritious meals with extra glucose / sugar. Allow child to eat what he or she likes.
- If child is vomiting, do <u>not</u> give Stemetil®, Largactil®, or any similar drugs, as these are toxic to the liver. Clear fluids only for 24 hours are usually all that will be needed. If vomiting persists, refer.
- Explain to parents that the child often feels better when jaundice appears. It will take one to two weeks to clear. Urine may remain dark for some weeks.
- Advise rest at home for the child, not necessarily in bed unless child does not want to be up and about.
- Advise parents about the mode of transmission of the disease (faecal–oral); child must eat from his or her own plate and utensils.
- Infectious precautions: Hygiene, hand washing, safe stool disposal.
- Notify the local health authorities of the home address, so that a visit can be made to enquire about water supplies and sewage disposal.
- Back to school when no longer clinically jaundiced.

Course and outcome

The vast majority of children recover in three to four weeks.

Note: Viral hepatitis is a notifiable disease.

Anicteric hepatitis (No jaundice)

Probably the most common form of viral hepatitis. Similar symptoms as in the pre-icteric form of the illness, but less severe. Seldom diagnosed in children unless liver function tests done, that is, when there are other cases in the area and hepatitis is suspected. Adults are generally immune because of antibodies present, the result of undiagnosed hepatitis in childhood.

Fulminant hepatitis (Acute liver failure)
Rarely the child may die from acute failure of the liver before jaundice appears, or it may follow an ordinary attack of jaundice, where the symptoms are progressive and are accompanied by confusion and drowsiness. At this stage, EEG is abnormal. There may be delirium and convulsions indicating involvement of the nervous system. The liver gets smaller, the child goes into coma and, in nearly all cases, dies of acute liver failure within days or weeks of the onset. An occasional recovery occurs, but there is no specific treatment available for the disease.

Prophylaxis with immunoglobulin

Hepatitis A
Most effective when pooled immunoglobulin given soon after contact, but has some effect any time before the onset of illness. Probably modifies rather than protects.
Dosage: Household exposure – 0,02–0,04 ml/kg
          Prolonged exposure – 0,03–0,06 ml/kg

Hepatitis B
Pooled immunoglobulin is ineffective. Hyperimmune immunoglobulin should be given within five days of exposure.

Hepatitis B vaccine
This is now part of the routine immunisation programme for infants. Vaccine plus hyperimmune immunoglobulin should be given to all infants born to a woman who is HBsAG positive.

Herpes simplex
See Ear, nose, throat, and mouth, p. 140.

Definition
Herpes simplex is a viral infection with a high recurrence rate, marked by latent periods and repeated, localised lesions consisting of painful blisters with crust formation.

Aetiology
The causative agent is Herpesvirus hominus types I and II (HVH I and II). HVH I is responsible for fever blisters, herpes stomatitis, herpetic lesions complicating eczema, aseptic meningitis in older children, and 10% of neonatal infections. HVH II is responsible for genital herpes and most

neonatal herpes infections acquired by passage through an infected birth canal.

Clinical course and findings
Primary herpes infections

Contact with HVH I usually occurs in the first five years of life. Most infections are subclinical. In about 10% of primary infections, obvious disease occurs.

- **Stomatitis:** This begins with fever and malaise for a week or more. Painful lesions occur on the mucous membranes. These start out as small blister-like lesions on the gums, tongue, throat, and anywhere else in the mouth. They soon break, leaving greyish-yellow ulcers. These lesions appear to have a white base and are very often misdiagnosed as thrush which does not have pain and fever. Tenderness and swelling of the submandibular lymph nodes are usually present. The gum lesions tend to bleed and are typical. Dehydration is an important complication due to the painful mouth.
- **Kerato-conjunctivitis:** HVH I may infect the eye causing kerato-conjunctivitis
- **Aseptic meningitis or encephalitis:** Both HVH I and II may rarely cause aseptic meningitis or encephalitis. There is a high fatality rate with neurological abnormalities in most of the survivors, if not diagnosed and treated early.
- **Herpes infection in the newborn infant:** In 90% of cases this is caused by HVH II due to spread after rupture of the membranes, or with passage through the birth canal during delivery. HVH infection may rarely be due to spread across the placenta. Occasionally infection of neonates may spread from nursing staff, or mothers with secondary herpes of the lips. HVH may cause a mild disease, but it mostly causes a severe infection affecting all organs. Generalised herpes is often fatal if not treated early.
- **Disseminated herpes infection:** Also occurs in malnourished infants, infants with AIDS or in measles with a high fatality rate.
- **Herpes-infected Eczema:** Occurs as widespread lesions on eczematous skin with a wide variation of severity.

Secondary herpes infection

Cold Sores: These occur in any patient who has had a previous primary herpes infection and has developed antibodies against HVH. The reactivated lesions are often at the mucocutaneous junctions, but can be anywhere on the skin or mucous membranes. The lesions are localised and painful but not accompanied by systemic reaction. Non-specific triggers such as sunburn, cold, fever, or emotional stress are responsible for reactivation. In children the lesions are usually on the lips. These are self-limiting and clear up in seven to ten days.

Diagnosis
- The clinical picture as described is often specific enough to make the diagnosis.
- Laboratory tests:
  - The vesicle fluid can be identified by electron microscopy in severe cases.
  - The virus can be cultured.

Treatment
- Treatment of gingivo-stomatitis:
  - Anti-fever drugs and analgesics may be necessary. Local anaesthetics such as lignocaine in tannic acid or Teejel® may relieve pain and thereby improve fluid and food intake. Sodium bicarbonate mouth washes are soothing.
  - Encourage fluid intake to prevent dehydration. Bland lukewarm fluids, for example milk, are best tolerated.
  - Keep the mouth clean. Antiseptic mouthwashes may be used in older children. Tube-feeding or intravenous fluids may be necessary in severe cases.
- Specific: Acyclovir intravenously may be needed in very severe cases or in children with immune supression including HIV/AIDS.
- Supportive therapy is of the utmost importance in severe cases.
- Kerato-conjunctivitis, aseptic meningitis, and neonatal herpes should be referred for treatment with acyclovir

Infectious mononucleosis (Glandular fever)
Definition
Glandular fever is an acute infectious disease characterised by malaise, irregular fever, sore throat, lymphadenopathy, and splenomegaly.

Aetiology
It is caused by the Epstein Barr (EB) virus of the herpes group of viruses.

Transmission
This is probably through saliva from person to person by close contact.

Incubation
The period probably varies from two to six weeks.

Isolation period
None.

Clinical course and findings
Prodomal: Slow and insidious onset.

Stage of advance: In children, this is often a mild disease with fever, lymphadenopathy, enlarged liver and spleen, and a sore throat. It may also be much more severe with an exudative pharyngo-tonsillitis. Jaundice may occur in about 4% of cases. A roseolar skin rash confined to the trunk may occur on the fourth to tenth day of illness. The disease may last from one to several weeks.

Complications
- Jaundice due to acute hepatitis.
- Aseptic meningitis occasionally.
- Myocarditis and pneumonia.
- Spontaneous or traumatic rupture of the enlarged spleen may occur.
- Glandular fever is rarely fatal.

Diagnosis
- The clinical picture is non-specific.
- Laboratory investigations include:
  - A full blood count looking for atypical lymphocytes. There is an increase in total mononuclear cells, monocytes and lymphocytes.
  - The Paul-Bunnell test. This often becomes positive late in the disease, and a rising titre is more important than an initial low positive titre. A negative Paul-Bunnell test does not exclude the diagnosis.
  - EB virus antibodies.

Treatment
There is no specific treatment.

Supportive
- Bed rest is usually advised to prevent rupture of the enlarged friable spleen in the acute phase of the disease.
- In severe pharyngo-tonsillitis, penicillin should be given to combat secondary infection. Do not give ampicillin, as 80% will develop a rash.

Prevention
No preventive measures are necessary.

Malaria
Definition
Malaria usually presents with repeated attacks of fever, malaise, chills and sweating, headache and, in 50% of cases, splenomegaly.

Aetiology
Malaria is a parasitic infection produced by one of four species of Plasmodium. *P. falciparum* malaria is the main type seen in southern Africa.

Transmission
This is through an infected female Anopheles mosquito. Sporozoites concentrate in the salivary glands of the mosquito, and are injected into humans when bitten.

Incubation period
Up to 12 days for *P. falciparum.*

Isolation period
None.

Clinical course and findings (In *P. falciparum* infection)
Stage of advance: A typical attack of malaria in children usually starts as a 'flu-like' illness with fever, tiredness, headaches, muscle pain and occasionally abdominal pain, diarrhoea, vomiting, and cough. The temperature is often intermittent and may be accompanied by profuse sweating. These spikes in temperature occur because of red blood cells rupturing and freeing the parasites into the blood stream. This haemolysis, when severe, can cause anaemia, jaundice, and blackwater fever (passing of free haemoglobin in the urine).

Complications
- Febrile convulsions.
- Anaemia and jaundice.
- Hypotension and shock.
- Cerebral malaria resulting in coma.
- Haemolysis may cause haemoglobinuria (blackwater fever), glomerulonephritis, nephrotic syndrome, and renal failure.

Diagnosis
• The above clinical picture in a person living in, or who has visited a malaria area is highly suggestive.
• A high index of suspicion is essential in making good early diagnoses of malaria.
• A definitive diagnosis can be made on a thick bloodsmear examination. Repeated smears taken during temperature spikes may be necessary.
• Serum antigen tests for malaria are rapid and accurate.

Treatment
Specific
(i) Oral quinine 10 mg/kg eight-hourly for seven days PLUS clindamycin 5 mg/kg eight-hourly for seven days or doxycycline (if over eight years of age) 4 mg/kg immediately then 2 mg/kg daily for seven days. The quinine tablets are very bitter but can be crushed and taken with jam or banana.
(ii) A combination of oral artemisinin-based drugs such as Coartem® taken immediately, then again at eight hours, followed by twice daily for the next two days. Dose: One tablet if 10–14 kg, two tablets if 15–24 kg, three tablets if 25–34 kg, and four tablets if 35 kg or more.

Most strains of malaria are now resistant to chloroquine alone or in combination with other drugs. Paracetamol is best for reducing the fever. Make sure the patient is taking enough fluids.

Severe malaria is usually treated with intravenous quinine PLUS doxy-cycline or clindamycin. Intravenous drugs must be started immediately and the patient referred to hospital urgently.

Supportive
• Anti-fever measures to prevent convulsions.
• Intravenous fluids for dehydration or renal failure.
• Blood transfusion may be needed for severe anaemia or circulatory collapse.

Prophylaxis
Malaria prophylaxis is needed by all who enter a malaria area (a region where malaria occurs). The risk of becoming infected by malaria is particularly high in the rainy season when mosquitoes are common. Full compliance is very important. However, no prophylaxis is 100% effective.

1. Malanil® (atovaquone plus proguanil) for children of 5 kg or more.
2. Mefloquine (Larium®) for children of 5 kg or more.
3. Doxycycline for older children (over eight years).

It is best for all children under five years, especially children under 5 kg, not to enter a malaria area as they are at high risk for severe infection. Chloroquine alone, chloroquine with proguanil, and Coartem® should not be used for prophylaxis.

Prevention
- Eradication of the mosquito by spraying of houses and breeding places for at least four consecutive years.
- Screens over doors and windows and sleeping nets over beds.
- Taking prophylactic treatment before entering malaria areas and completing prophylaxis after leaving the area.
- Wear long sleeves and trousers with shoes and socks in evenings and early morning. Topical repellents will help.
- Use insecticide impregnated bed-nets.

Measles
Definition
Measles is an acute severe illness which is highly infectious. It has a prodromal phase followed by a typical dusty-red, blotchy maculo-papular rash (morbilliform). Due to the severity of the illness and the immune suppression it causes, it has many serious complications.

Aetiology
It is caused by the measles virus.

Transmission
This is by droplet spread or direct contact with secretions of the nose and throat of infected persons. Measles is one of the most readily transmitted infectious diseases. The child is most infectious to others during the prodromal phase, often before the diagnosis is made.

Incubation period
Medium (seven to 14 days; usually ten to 12 days).

Isolation period
For five days after appearance of the rash.

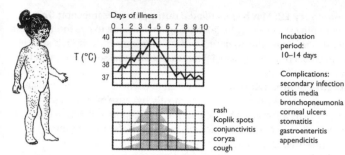

Figure 10.1 Clinical course of measles

Clinical course and findings

Prodromal phase

This may last three to seven days, but is usually four days. The first symptoms are a runny nose, fever, conjunctivitis, and coughing. Koplik spots appear 24–48 hours before the rash. These are small white spots on a red base inside the cheeks, usually opposite the lower molars, but may occur on gums and inside lips as well.

Stage of advance

The maculo-papular rash starts behind the ears and on the forehead and spreads downwards. It takes about three days to reach the feet, at which point it starts to fade. Fever is high and lasts for four to five days after the appearance of the rash. There may be skin pigmentation (staining) and desquamation after the rash disappears.

Complications

These tend to be both more common and severe in malnourished children.

- **Pneumonia**: This is usually viral pneumonitis occurring in the first few days after the rash appears. It is caused either by the measles virus itself or by the herpes or adenovirus. Pneumonia may occur later and is then due to secondary bacterial infection. In malnourished children, staphylococci and Gram-negative bacilli are often responsible and should be treated vigorously.
- **Laryngotracheobronchitis**: This presents with dry, brassy cough and stridor, and can be so severe in young infants that intubation is required.
- **Otitis media**: This is very common.

- **Pulmonary TB**: May be reactivated during measles infection. The tuberculin skin test may be falsely negative for one to two months after measles infection due to depressed cellular immunity. If TB is strongly suspected, commence with TB treatment and reassess the patient in two months' time.
- **Kerato-conjunctivitis**: This may result in corneal ulceration, causing a cloudy cornea when healed. It is mostly because of secondary herpes virus infection. May be complicated by vitamin A deficiency in malnourished children. Do not use steroids. Refer for treatment.
- **Encephalitis**: This is a serious complication, often fatal or with residual brain damage.
- **Gastroenteritis**.
- **Oral thrush and / or oral herpes**.

Diagnosis

- **Clinical**: The clinical picture is usually typical enough to make the diagnosis possible even before the rash appears. This is especially so when a history of contact with measles is available and Koplik spots are seen.
- **Laboratory**: Although the virus can be cultured, it is seldom necessary or of practical value.

Treatment

Specific: No specific treatment is available.

Supportive:
- Anti-fever measures are often necessary.
- Plenty of fluids must be given to combat dehydration.
- Eye and mouth hygiene.
- The child should be checked frequently for complications.
- Vitamin A 200 000 units orally daily for two days.
- While uncomplicated cases may be nursed at home, small infants, malnourished children, and those with complications should be treated in a hospital with isolation facilities.

Prevention

Measles can be prevented through active immunisation which must be carried out in all children. All unimmunised children who are six months and older should be immunised on admission to a paediatric ward. In an exposed and unimmunised child, the infection can be aborted if vaccine is given within 12 hours of exposure. Passive immunity lasting for four weeks can be achieved by giving gammaglobulin 0,25 ml/kg IM within seven days of exposure. Two ml of measles-specific human immunoglobulin will have the same effect.

Note: Measles is a notifiable disease and presently all cases of suspected measles must be reported to your provincial office. You will be requested to obtain blood and urine specimens. The provincial office with your help will organise an outbreak response.

Meningococcal infection
Definition
This is an acute bacterial disease characterised by sudden onset of fever, headache, nausea, vomiting, stiff neck or bulging fontanelle, and frequently a purpuric rash.

Aetiology
It is caused by an intracellular Gram-negative coccus, *Neisseria meningitides.*

Transmission
By direct contact, including droplet spread. The incidence of clinical disease after contact is low, but with a very high rate of healthy carriers.

Incubation period
Short (seven days).

Isolation period
For two days after starting treatment.

Clinical course and findings
Meningococcal infection can present as two separate clinical entities:
• Meningitis.
• Septicaemia.

Meningitis
Prodromal phase: None.
Stage of advance: The onset is usually abrupt with fever, headache, and irritability. This is followed by signs of meningeal irritation, for example neck stiffness, positive Kernig's sign, etc. Evidence of raised intracranial pressure may be present, with nausea, vomiting, and a bulging or tense fontanelle (when open). A petechial rash develops in about 30% of cases.

Complications:
- Meningococcal septicaemia (see below).
- Pneumonia.
- Arthritis.
- Central nervous system:
  - Hydrocephalus.
  - Cranial nerve palsies.
  - Mental retardation.
  - Subdural effusions.
  - Deafness.
  - Blindness.
  - Epilepsy.

Meningococcal septicaemia
Prodromal phase: Absent.
Stage of advance: The onset is abrupt, with the appearance of a rash, fever, and signs of circulatory collapse, for example rapid weak pulse. This may go on to irreversible shock. Other accompanying signs may be headache, shivering, abdominal pain, vomiting, and diarrhoea. The rash tends to be progressive, starting as petechiae and going on to purpura and to ecchymoses. Bleeding into the adrenals produces severe and usually irreversible shock and is known as the Waterhouse-Friderichsen Syndrome. Meningitis is often but not always present. If septicaemia is not treated early and energetically, the outcome is usually fatal.

Diagnosis of meningococcal infection
Clinical: The diagnosis is basically clinical. Any ill child with purpura must be suspected of having meningococcal infection and treated as such until proven otherwise.

Laboratory:
- On lumbar puncture, the cerebrospinal fluid shows the picture of a septic meningitis. Gram-negative diplococci may be seen on Gram staining of the cerebrospinal fluid. In septicaemia, the CSF may be normal, but lumbar puncture is contraindicated because of the associated cerebral oedema and danger of coning.
- Skin scrapings of purpuric lesions can be stained or cultured for meningococci.
- Blood culture may be positive.
- Buffy coat stains.

Treatment
Specific: IV antibiotic therapy must be started immediately. As meningococcal septicaemia is an emergency, start treatment with IV cefotaxime 50 mg/kg per dose six-hourly as soon as the rash is seen. As soon as possible, give dexamethasone 0,15 mg/kg per dose six-hourly.

In a clinic or other situation where the diagnosis is suspected and the patient is waiting for transfer to hospital, it is essential to begin treatment as above while waiting. Use the IM route if IV is not possible. In an emergency, if cephalosporins are not available, use IV penicillin G 125,000 U/kg per dose six-hourly plus chloramphenicol 25 mg/kg per dose six-hourly.

Do not do a lumbar puncture.

Supportive treatment:
- Give fluids intravenously.
- Treat shock appropriately.
- Heparin or steroids may be given in hospital under medical supervision in cases of meningococcal septicaemia. This is to treat the disseminated intravascular coagulopathy.

Prevention
Household contacts should be given rifampicin (capsules 600 mg and 150 mg; syrup 100 mg/5 ml).

Adults: 600 mg 12-hourly for two days.
Children: 10 mg/kg 12-hourly for two days (less than
            5 kg: 5 mg/kg 12-hourly for two days).

Note: Meningococcal infection is a notifiable disease in South Africa. The provincial office must be notified. This will help with an appropriate and rapid response to the outbreak.

Mumps
Definition
Mumps is an acute viral disease characterised by fever, swelling, and tenderness of one or more of the salivary glands, usually the parotids.

Aetiology
Mumps is caused by a virus from the myxovirus group. Transmission is by droplet spread or by direct contact with saliva from an infected person.

Incubation period
Long: 14–21 days.

Isolation period
Until swelling has subsided completely.

Clinical course and findings
Prodromal phase: Usually absent, but an occasional patient may present with fever, sore throat, and pain on chewing before the swelling appears. Stage of advance: Painful swelling of one or both parotids occurs. In 10% of cases, the swelling starts in the submandibular glands. The parotid glands enlarge in the same axis as the ear, lifting the lower part of the ear.

Complications:
- The testes or ovaries may be involved causing severe pain, but this is rare in children before puberty.
- Deafness is a rare complication.
- Pancreatitis is a rare complication and causes severe abdominal pain with vomiting and sometimes diarrhoea.

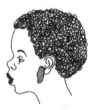

Parotid gland normally impalpable

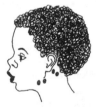

Normal cervical nodes

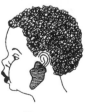

Mumps

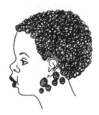

Cervical lymphadenopathy

Figure 10.2 Parotid gland swelling compared with lymph nodes

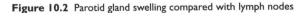

- Mumps meningoencephalitis may occur, usually with an uncomplicated course and full recovery.

Diagnosis
Clinical: The diagnosis on the clinical picture usually presents no problem.

Laboratory:
- A rise in mumps virus antibody titre is an indication of a recent infection.
- The virus can be cultured when necessary.

Treatment
Specific: None.
Supportive:
- Analgesics and antipyretics should be given as required.
- Oral hygiene is necessary because of decreased flow of saliva.
- A fluid diet may be necessary in the acute phase.

Prevention
The Mumps-Measles-Rubella (MMR) vaccine provides good immunity.

Poliomyelitis
Definition
Poliomyelitis is a viral disease which may cause damage to motor cells of the spinal cord and brainstem, resulting in asymmetrical weakness or paralysis of the muscles that are supplied by the affected segments of the cord.

Aetiology
Poliomyelitis is caused by three types of polio virus, namely types I, II, and III.

Transmission
By direct contact with pharyngeal secretions or faeces.

Incubation period
Medium (seven to 14 days).

Isolation period

In hospital for seven to ten days. Isolation has little value in the home environment because the spread of infection is greatest in the prodromal phase.

Clinical course and findings

Prodromal phase: In this stage, the virus is multiplying in the pharynx and gastro-intestinal tract, and the patient presents with a flu-like disease. These symptoms usually disappear within two days. If the disease does not progress any further, this is called abortive poliomyelitis and is usually only recognised under epidemic conditions.

Stage of advance: The virus multiplies in the central nervous system, and the patient complains of headache, anorexia, and fever. Signs of meningeal irritation, muscular pains, and tenderness develop. This may clear up in six to eight days, leaving no damage. This is called non-paralytic poliomyelitis.

In more severe cases, paralysis begins on the third or fourth day of the illness but rarely occurs after the fever has subsided. In infants and young children, the paralysis may be the first sign of the illness. The paralysis is of a lower motor neurone lesion type, featuring flaccid weakness with an asymmetrical distribution. Involvement may be:

- Spinal with paralysis in the limbs or respiratory muscles.
- Central (brainstem) with cranial nerve palsies or respiratory or circulatory centre disturbances.

Complications:

- Respiratory failure: This should be carefully watched for and treated with intermittent positive pressure ventilation.
- Circulatory collapse.
- Permanent paralysis with resulting disability.

Diagnosis

Clinical:

This may be difficult until paralysis occurs, except in epidemic situations with a high index of suspicion.

Laboratory:

- The virus can be cultured from the faeces.
- A rise in antibody titre occurs in active poliomyelitis.

- A lumbar puncture should not be done if poliomyelitis is strongly suspected, as local trauma may result in increased paralysis in that area. For the same reason, exercise and IM injections should be avoided. The cerebrospinal fluid shows the picture of aseptic meningitis.

Treatment
Specific treatment is not available.

Supportive:
- Bed rest is essential in the acute phase, as activity is inclined to worsen the paralysis.
- Intermittent positive pressure respiration should be available when necessary.
- Physiotherapy and rehabilitation for patients with permanent paralysis.

Prevention
Live virus trivalent (types I, II, and III) vaccine is very effective, and should be given to all infants and children to prevent a crippling and sometimes fatal disease. In addition, trivalent (types I to III) vaccine is given to all newborn infants on discharge from hospital or clinic. Vaccination against poliomyelitis is not compulsory in South Africa.

Note: Poliomyelitis is a notifiable disease. As we are trying to have a polio-free world, there is an active surveillance process in this country; thus, please contact the provincial office for all cases of acute flaccid paralysis.

Rabies
Definition
Rabies is an almost invariably fatal acute encephalitis.

Aetiology
It is caused by the rabies virus.

Transmission
Rabies is primarily a disease of animals and is transmitted to humans by means of virus-laden saliva from a rabid animal (e.g. dog, cat, jackal, mongoose, bat, etc.) being introduced by a bite or lick.

Incubation period
20–90 days or longer.

Isolation period
None.

Clinical course and findings
Onset begins with a sense of apprehension, headache, fever, malaise, and indefinite sensory changes often referred to the site of the bite. This is followed by agitation, delirium, hyperactivity, inability to swallow, and convulsions. Paralysis occurs in 20% of cases. Coma and death are the usual outcomes.

Diagnosis
Clinical: In sporadic cases, the diagnosis may be difficult on the clinical picture alone. Due to the long incubation period, the bite may have been forgotten by the time symptoms appear. Paralytic rabies (20%) may be misdiagnosed as Guillain-Barre syndrome or polio. The diagnosis is usually made on the abnormal behaviour and symptoms of the patient.

Laboratory:
- Rabies virus can be cultured. This is done mostly from the neurological tissues of the rabid animal.
- A rise in antibody titre against rabies supports the diagnosis.

Treatment
- Specific: No specific treatment is available after onset of symptoms.
- Supportive treatment should be given as necessary, for example for convulsions, respiratory failure, etc.

Prevention
- Wash wound thoroughly with soap and water as soon as possible. Apply Betadine®, Cetrimide® or iodine. A deep, penetrating wound should be cleaned surgically. Give tetanus toxoid.
- In a rabies endemic area, the patient should be referred to the local authorities for further management.
- Infection may be prevented by administration of human anti-rabies immunoglobulin 20 IU/kg, half IM and half infiltrated around the wound as soon after being bitten as possible, followed by active immunisation with human diploid cell rabies vaccine.
- Personnel at risk from rabies can be immunised with rabies vaccine.
Note: Rabies is a notifiable disease.

Roseola infantum
Definition
An acute viral illness presenting with a high fever and rash.

Aetiology
Herpes 6 virus.

Incubation period
Unknown.

Isolation period
None.

Clinical presentation
- Presents with a high fever.
- Macular erythematous rash on trunk appears as the fever falls.
- The illness resolves spontaneously in a few days.

Complications
- Pyrexial convulsions.

Treatment
- Supportive, with antipyretics.

Rubella (German measles)
Definition
Rubella is a mild and usually uncomplicated febrile infectious disease, characterised by enlargement of the suboccipital lymph nodes and a fine maculo-papular rash which itches slightly.

Although the illness is mild in children, the condition is significant because it causes serious damage to the embryo in early pregnancy.

Aetiology
It is caused by the rubella virus.

Transmission
The disease is generally spread through secretions of the upper respiratory tract. In congenital rubella, it is acquired transplacentally and the virus can be found in pharyngeal secretions, urine, faeces, and blood of an infected newborn infant.

Incubation period
Long (14–21 days).

Isolation period
Pregnant women who may be suseptible to rubella should keep away from an infected individual for at least 14 days after the rash has faded.

Clinical course and findings
Prodromal phase: In children there are often no prodromal symptoms and the presenting sign is the rash. In teenagers and adults, pyrexia, malaise, and sore throat (catarrhal symptoms) precede the rash.

Stage of advance: The rash starts with discrete, fine, pink macules on the face spreading to the trunk, arms, and legs. It becomes more confluent and typically fades in one part as it appears in another. The rash only occurs over a few days. Lymphadenopathy is a constant feature of rubella. Classically the suboccipital and posterior cervical nodes are enlarged, but occasionally other groups are affected.

Complications:
- Encephalitis rarely occurs.
- Arthritis may develop, usually in female adults, but is uncommon in children.
- Congenital rubella syndrome (see p. 109).

Diagnosis
- The clinical picture is usually sufficiently characteristic to make the diagnosis.
- Laboratory: The virus can be cultured or a rise in antibody titre shown. Pregnant women exposed to rubella virus must have antibody titres done. If the initial titre is high, maternal immunity can be presumed and there is minimal risk to the fetus. In the case of a rising titre in early pregnancy, medical abortion should be considered.

Treatment
- No specific treatment is available.
- Supportive treatment if necessary.

Prevention
Rubella vaccine should be given to all children, especially pre-pubertal girls due to the danger of congenital rubella syndrome. MMR is usually used in infants. Natural wild virus infection gives life-long immunity against rubella, while rubella vaccine does not seem to give as high or as prolonged a rise in antibody titre.

Tetanus
Definition
Tetanus is characterised by muscle rigidity and painful muscle spasms.

Aetiology
It is caused by the toxin of the anaerobic *Clostridium tetani.*

Transmission
Tetanus spores are introduced into the body during injury, usually a penetrating wound contaminated with soil or faeces, but also through burns or trivial wounds. Neonatal tetanus occurs through infection of the umbilical cord stump.

Incubation period
Medium (four days to three weeks; average ten days). In general, the longer the incubation period, the milder the disease.

Isolation period
None.

Clinical course and findings
Neonatal tetanus:
The first signs are usually difficulty in sucking and trismus (clenched jaw). This is followed by rigidity of the abdominal wall muscles and generalised spasms.

Older children:
Present with muscle rigidity, followed by generalised painful spasms. Sometimes the original injury may already have been forgotten when symptoms appear.

Complications:
- The fatality rate is still high. In survivors, recovery is complete.
- Aspiration pneumonia.
- Apnoea and hypoxia develop during prolonged muscle spasms.

Diagnosis

This is on the clinical picture. No laboratory tests are available. Tetanus bacilli can be cultured anaerobically, but are difficult to recover from the wound.

Treatment

- Give Procaine penicillin 100 000 units IM twice daily for five days to prevent further toxin production.
- Give 500 units human tetanus immunoglobulin IM in a neonate and 2 000 units to an older child.
- If practical, transfer to specialised unit immediately for intensive care. Paralysis and ventilation may be needed.
- Supportive treatment includes IV fluids, nasogastric feeding, and wound cleaning where applicable.

Prevention

Neonatal tetanus:
- Immunisation of pregnant mothers at antenatal clinics in areas with a high incidence of neonatal tetanus.
- Routine cord care with surgical spirits.
- Educate mothers in cord hygiene.

Older children:
- Immunise against tetanus. When fully immunised, protection lasts at least five years.
- Give tetanus toxoid to all children with contaminated wounds.
- Surgical cleaning of deep wounds, antibiotics, and additional 250 units human anti-tetanus immunoglobulin in suspicious or severe wounds.

Note: Tetanus is a notifiable disease.

Tick-bite fever

Definition

Tick-bite fever is characterised by sudden onset of fever, headache, chills, and conjunctivitis, followed three days later by a maculo-papular rash.

Aetiology
It is a rickettsial disease caused by *Rickettsia rickettsii*.

Transmission
This is through the bite of an infected tick after several hours of attachment. Infected ticks are prevalent everywhere in South Africa, with a higher concentration in some areas.

Incubation period
Medium (seven to ten days).

Isolation period
None.

Clinical course and findings
Prodromal stage: Precedes the rash by three to four days. It consists of fever, chills, headache, and injected conjunctiva, causing photophobia. If looked for carefully, a primary lesion at the site of the tick bite can usually be found. This consists of an ulcer with a black centre and red areola (eschar). Regional lymphadenopathy is usually present.

Stage of advance: A maculo-papular rash, often haemorrhagic, may develop on the third to fourth day. It frequently involves the palms and soles as well. Abdominal pain, arthritis, hepatitis, and other organ involvement may occur.

Complications: Fatalities are rare in children, even without treatment.

Diagnosis
- Clinical: The diagnosis should be made on the clinical picture, especially if an eschar and local adenopathy can be found.
- Laboratory: The Weil-Felix test is positive, with a rise in titre being more specific.

Treatment
- Specific: Tetracycline (doxycycline) by mouth is the antibiotic of choice. It usually settles the temperature within 48 hours. Tetracycline should generally not be given to children under seven years of age, but one course should not damage the tooth enamel.
- Supportive: Analgesics should be given.

Prevention
- Avoid tick-infested areas where possible.
- Remove ticks from the body carefully without squeezing.
- Vaccines are available, but seldom necessary.

Tuberculosis

Definition

Tuberculosis is a chronic bacterial infection which can affect all organs of the body, with pulmonary TB being the most common.

Aetiology

The causative organisms are:
- *Mycobacterium tuberculosis:* The human tubercle bacillus which is responsible for most pulmonary tuberculosis.
- *Mycobacterium bovis:* Which is mainly found in the milk of TB-infected cattle. This can cause intestinal or pulmonary TB in humans.
- The transmission of *M. tuberculosis* is from person to person through airborne spread. *M. bovis* is ingested through drinking unpasteurised milk. Children are almost always infected by being coughed on by tuberculous adults who have millions of TB bacilli in their sputum. The state of a child's immunity is a key factor in determining the extent to which the infection progresses. TB may, therefore, present in any condition that suppresses the cellular immunity of the patient. The common causes of this are kwashiorkor, HIV/AIDS, post-measles or pertussis; patients on medications such as steroids or cytotoxics are also vulnerable.

Background to prevention

Tuberculosis is one of the greatest health problems of under-developed countries. Its transmission is by droplet spread from the sputum of affected adults. In overcrowded housing, cramped workplaces, and transport systems where people are crushed together, the chances of transmission are much greater. The ability of an infected adult or child to produce a satisfactory immune response to the disease is seriously affected by undernutrition and the presence of immune-depressing conditions such as AIDS and measles. In addition, the ability of the health services to detect, diagnose, and treat cases depends on how well they are organised and how much cooperation they have from the community.

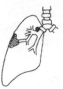
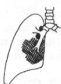

a. Primary Complex   b. TB pneumonia   c. TB effusion

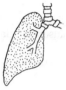

d. Miliary TB   e. Partial obstruction   f. Obstruction
with hyperinflation   with collapse

Figure 10.3 Range of pulmonary TB

Pathology

A small focus of infection develops in the lung, with subsequent infection and enlargement of the associated lymph nodes at the hilum of the lung, or those alongside the trachea. This is known as the primary complex, and its development takes about six weeks.

At this stage, the tuberculin test becomes positive and will always remain so. If the child's immunity is good, he or she recovers and the lungs do not become further affected. On the other hand, if immunity is poor, the infection will spread from the enlarged lymph nodes into the surrounding lung or along the airways to other parts of the lung. This is 'progressive primary' or full-blown pulmonary TB in children.

Latent or dormant TB infection from years before may be reactivated to give progressive pulmonary TB, especially if immunity is depressed by undernutrition, measles or HIV infection.

Isolation period

Although patients are seldom isolated, they stay infective for as long as tubercle bacilli are discharged into the sputum. Due to the different nature of the disease in children as compared to adults, adults are much more infectious than children. After starting treatment, the sputum usually becomes sterile within a few weeks.

Common presentations of the various forms of TB
Pulmonary
- Asymptomatic: This is the case with the primary complex stage, although even progressive primary TB may show very few symptoms.
- Poor weight gain or even weight loss.
- Chronic cough.
- Severe respiratory distress and wheezing: This is caused by enlarged lymph nodes compressing the main bronchi.
- The production of sputum and haemopysis are typical in adult TB, but are not major features of childhood TB.

Diagnosis is by tuberculin skin testing, chest X-ray and, in certain cases, testing the sputum for AFBs. The sputum is often negative in children despite the disease being strongly present.

TB of the cervical lymph nodes
Cervical glandular tuberculosis presents with chronically enlarged neck nodes which are non-tender, firm, and often matted together. Infection reaches these nodes from the tonsils where the TB organism first gains entry. If left untreated, they break down and chronic sinus formation may occur.

Diagnosis is by biopsy.

TB meningitis (TBM)
TB meningitis has a slow and deceptive onset. In the earliest stages, there may be personality changes, lethargy, and headaches. In later stages, symptoms include irritability, anorexia, vomiting, and fever going on to drowsiness, loss of consciousness, and finally coma. A high level of suspicion is essential when treating any child with these features. Early diagnosis is critical because the quality of survival depends on the stage of first diagnosis. Many children who survive TBM have residual disabilities such as deafness, cerbral palsy, mental retardation or epilepsy.

Diagnosis is by means of lumbar puncture. Even with mild symptoms, the CSF will be abnormal.

Spinal tuberculosis

TB infection of the vertebral bodies at first causes backache. The affected vertebrae eventually collapse, with compression of the spinal cord. This affects the innervation of the legs, bladder, and bowel. An obvious hunch-back or 'gibus' may become visible. Chronic back pain and / or gibbus in a child need(s) urgent attention.

Diagnosis is by means of tuberculin testing and X-ray of the spine.

Diagnosis of tuberculosis

Clinical:

A high index of suspicion is essential, as TB is a great mimic. There are two conditions that are very often associated with TB and therefore are useful in its diagnosis, namely phlyctenular conjunctivitis and erythema nodosum.

Phlyctenular conjunctivitis

- This condition is a hypersensitivity reaction to tuberculo-protein in the conjunctiva of the eye and may occur at all stages of activity of a primary complex.
- Clinical: The lesion begins as a small vesicle or ulcerated nodule situated at the corneo-conjunctival junction (limbus). Injected blood-vessels radiate outwards from the lesion and the whole conjunctiva is inflamed. There is extreme photophobia with tearing. The eye is kept tightly closed, and there is resistance to the examination of the eye. The lesion may lead to ulceration of the cornea. Because of the hypersensitivity, only one tuberculin unit and not the normal five should be used for skin-testing, as skin ulceration may occur at the testing site and the eye lesion may be aggravated. It may be reasonable to assume a positive tuberculin test when a phlycten is present.
- Treatment: Refer the patient to an ophthalmologist for treatment, as steroid preparations may be necessary. The patient's TB must also be investigated.
- There is a tendency to relapse.

Erythema nodosum

- There are warm, swollen, tender erythematous nodules in the skin over the shins which come out in crops and fade, looking like bruises. TB is only one of many known causes but should always be investigated in any child showing these lesions.

Tuberculin skin testing

Infection with the TB bacillus induces a hypersensitivity in the patient which can be used to assist diagnosis of TB. The Tuberculin test is done by injecting tuberculoprotein into the skin and observing a reaction 48-72 hours later. Tuberculin sensitivity takes six weeks to develop, so testing early on in the infection will give a false-negative result.

A tuberculin test should be performed in any child suspected of having contracted TB. This would mean testing all children admitted to hospital, as well as any child with an unexplained illness who visits the outpatient department or the clinic.

The three common forms of tuberculin testing are the Mantoux, the Heaf, and the Tine tests. The Mantoux test is usually used.

The Mantoux test

0,1 ml of purified protein derivative (PPD) containing five tuberculin units is injected intracutaneously by convention on the left forearm. This should form a wheal about 7-8 mm in diameter. If a wheal is not produced, the injection has been given subcutaneously and should be repeated. Read the results in 72 hours, and measure the maximum diameter of induration as felt with the finger with a millimetre rule. The surrounding halo of erythema is not important.

Interpretation:
- 0-4 mm is a negative result.
- 5-9 mm is doubtful positive. It could be produced by BCG given previously or infection with atypical mycobacteria.
- 10 mm or more is positive. It could be produced by recent BCG or active or recent tuberculosis. Further investigations, for example chest X-ray and erythrocyte sedimentation rate (ESR), are now necessary.

The Tine test

This consists of a disposable unit with four prongs coated with dried PPD. The test is done by removing the protective cap, stretching the skin of the forearm after cleansing, and pressing the four prongs into the skin and holding for two to three seconds. The area of induration around the four prong marks is measured and recorded at 48-72 hours.

Interpretation:
- Grade I: A reaction of less than 2 mm is negative.
- Grade II: 2 mm or more is doubtful.

- Grade III: Fusion of two or more papules is a positive reaction.
- Grade IV: Fusion of all four puncture sites with central induration with or without ulceration constitutes a strongly positive reaction.

The significance of tuberculin test results:

- A negative test indicates that, so long as one of the causes of a false negative test is not present, the child has not been infected with *M. tuberculosis*, and needs BCG immunisation.
- A doubtful test means that the child probably has not been infected with *M. tuberculosis* and does not need immunisation.
- A positive test means that the child is now or has in the past been infected with *M. tuberculosis*.

Causes of false negative TB skin testing results:

- If the test is done incorrectly.
- If it is done within less than six weeks of the primary infection.
- In the presence of miliary or overwhelming tuberculous infection.
- If the child has HIV/AIDS.
- In the presence of malnutrition.
- If it is done within six weeks of measles or pertussis infection.
- In children on steroid or other immunosuppressive treatment.

Treatment of tuberculosis
Specific drug regimes

These vary in different regions of southern Africa. It is important to follow the official policy of the area in which the patient lives. Policies change from time to time, depending on economics, the discovery of new drugs, and the emergence of drug resistant strains of tubercle bacilli. Contact your local TB official for the most up-to-date guidelines on treatment.

Dosage

- Isoniazid (INH) 15–20 mg/kg/day in a single daily dose (maximum 300 mg/day).
- Ethionamide 10–20 mg/kg/day in a single daily dose (maximum 750 mg/day).
- Rifampicin 10–20 mg/kg/day in a single daily dose (maximum 600 mg/day).
- Pyrazinamide 30 mg/kg/day in a single daily dose (maximum 2 g/day).

The current regimens for pulmonary TB or primary complex disease involve the use of four drugs (multi-drug regimen) for 120 daily doses.

Breastfed babies of mothers with tuberculosis should stay on the breast, provided they are given INH 8 mg/kg/day once daily for three months, and the mother is treated at the same time. BCG is given to these babies once the course of INH is completed and the mother has been cured. INH administration to the baby must be stopped for at least 24 hours before BCG is given, as it will kill the BCG bacillus.

If tuberculosis is diagnosed early in pregnancy, drug treatment given to the mother should not produce congenital abnormalities in the baby. Streptomycin given to a pregnant mother, however, may cause congenital nerve deafness in the baby and should not be used.

Supportive treatment
- Attention to nutrition is very important.
- Treatment of anaemia and any intercurrent infection is essential.

Management of patients after skin testing
- All children under the age of five years with a positive skin test, but no clinical or X-ray sign of disease, are given a short course of treatment to prevent the further progress of the disease, especially later in adulthood (it is now believed that most adult TB is reactivated disease from childhood). These patients are notifiable to the local health authority as 'positive tuberculin reaction under five years of age'. The specific regimen varies. At present, it is Rifampicin and INH for three months.
- If a TB contact has a positive skin test, proceed as above. If the skin test is negative, give INH for two to three months and repeat the skin test. If it is positive, proceed as above. If it is negative again, stop treatment and give BCG.

Prevention
In line with what has been said above, rehousing programmes to replace overcrowded informal settlements are essential. Employment and social welfare programmes need to be improved to provide adequate nutrition for all. A well-organised primary health care system will prevent measles and other infectious disease, will work towards controlling AIDS, and will have an active TB programme integrated into its range of services. Some aspects of this programme would be:
- The case finding and treatment of adult cases with open infectious TB (the most important aspect of prevention).
- Household contacts of open cases need to be investigated, and any children should be given a tuberculin test and X-rayed if positive.

- All babies must be immunised with BCG at birth. This should be repeated at any time when a negative tuberculin reaction is found.

Typhoid
Definition
Typhoid is a systemic infectious disease characterised by fever, malaise, anorexia, and splenomegaly.

Aetiology
It is caused by *Salmonella typhi*.

Transmission
This is by ingestion of contaminated food or water by either patients or carriers. Poor sanitation predisposes the spread of the infection. The condition often occurs in epidemics due to a typhoid carrier contaminating a food or water source, but it also occurs in isolated cases.

Incubation period
Medium (one to three weeks, usually two weeks).

Isolation period
Patients should be isolated until three consecutive stool cultures taken 24 hours apart after stopping treatment are negative.

Clinical course and findings
Prodromal stage: None.
Stage of advance: Younger children may present with a fever for which no obvious clinical cause can be found. A blood culture at this early stage will always be positive for *S. typhi*. The older child commonly presents with persistent fever, headaches, abdominal pain, and coughing. There is more often constipation than diarrhoea. Further into the course of the illness there may be drowsiness, abdominal distension, bradycardia, and epistaxis. Splenomegaly is found in about a third of cases. In young children, there may be vomiting and diarrhoea which may be bloodstained in addition to the fever. Typhoid may also present as an encephalopathy with meningism, delirium, convulsions, and coma. Sometimes it may present as an acute septicaemia with drowsiness, shock, and jaundice. Rose spots, which usually appear on the trunk on the fifth to eighth day, are seldom seen in children.

Complications:
- Ulceration of Peyer's patches in the small intestine can result in perforation of the bowel and peritonitis.
- Neurological complications consist of convulsions, peripheral neuritis, hemiplegia, and encephalopathy.
- Bronchopneumonia.
- Hepatitis and jaundice.
- Myocarditis.
- Osteomyelitis and arthritis.

Diagnosis
The clinical picture is often non-specific, and the diagnosis must be confirmed with laboratory investigations.

Laboratory:
- Blood, urine, and faeces should be cultured for typhoid bacilli. The blood culture is usually positive early in the disease, while faeces and urine become positive in the second week of the illness.
- The Widal agglutination test usually becomes positive (1:320 or more) after ten days.

Treatment
Treatment should be started on suspicion without waiting for laboratory results, but after specimens are collected.

Specific:
- There is extensive resistance by the tyhpoid organism to a number of antibiotics. At present ciprofloxacin is the preferred antibiotic for typhoid fever while ceftriaxone is an acceptable alternative.

Supportive:
- Bed rest in the acute phase to prevent perforation. Be careful of transferring and transporting these patients.
- Antipyretics and fluid therapy may be necessary.
- Surgery is necessary for bowel perforation.

Prevention
- Good sanitation and purification of water supply are essential.
- Carriers should be identified and treated. If treatment is ineffective, carriers should not be allowed to handle food for public consumption.

- A vaccine (TAB) against typhoid is available, but is only used for people at high risk of exposure.

Note: Typhoid is a notifiable disease.

Whooping cough (Pertussis)
Definition
Pertussis is an acute bacterial disease involving the trachea, bronchi, and bronchioles.

Aetiology
The causative organism is *Bordetella pertussis*. (A similar 'whooping cough syndrome' is caused by other viral infections.)

Transmission
This is from person to person through direct contact or droplet spread. Patients are most infective during the catarrhal phase.

Incubation period
Medium (seven to 14 days).

Isolation period
For two days after starting treatment with erythromycin.

Clinical course and findings
Prodromal phase: The prodromal catarrhal phase usually lasts from seven to ten days. Only during this stage will the use of antibiotics have any effect on the subsequent course of the disease.

Stage of advance: Paroxysms of coughing develop, followed by the typical inspiratory whoop, and often followed by vomiting of clear mucus or food. Whooping cough may occur in neonates and infants under six months, as there is no transfer of immunity from the mother. Young infants present with severe pneumonia, apnoeic attacks with cyanosis, and sometimes convulsions. Once the cough develops, it may last for several weeks or months. The cough and whoop may sometimes recur with the next unrelated upper respiratory tract infection.

Complications:
- Epistaxis and sub-conjunctival haemorrhages are frequently seen.

Haemoptysis and facial purpura are due to the violence of the coughing. No treatment is necessary.

- Respiratory system: Persistent pneumonia or collapse of one or more lobes of the lung may occur. Bronchiectasis and pneumothorax are other complications. Pulmonary tuberculosis may be reactivated after pertussis infection.
- Repeated vomiting may result in dehydration and malnutrition. Re-feeding directly after a vomiting spell is often retained.
- Rectal prolapse may occur in malnourished children with whooping cough because of the increased intra-abdominal pressure during coughing.
- Neurological complications: The severe coughing episodes may lead to hypoxia resulting in cerebral oedema or, more rarely, haemorrhage.
- The younger the child, the greater the risk of complications and death.

Diagnosis

Clinical: Once the typical whoop is present, the clinical diagnosis is not difficult. This is often absent in small babies. Other conditions which give the same type of coughing are viral infections, tuberculous nodes, broncho-pneumonia, bronchitis, and a foreign body.

Laboratory investigations are not always helpful. *Bordetella pertussis* may be cultured from throat swabs, especially in the early stages of the disease. A full blood count may show a marked lymphocytosis with pertussis lymphocytes.

Treatment

Specific: Treatment with erythromycin for 14 days is used to stop the progress of the disease and to make the child non-infectious. Once the typical cough occurs, treatment with erythromycin does not change the clinical picture, although it does stop further spread of the infection to contacts.

Supportive:
- Coughing is difficult to control. A cough suppressant such as Nitepax® can be tried. Phenobarbitone in small doses or Aterax® are given in an attempt to control or lessen the paroxysms of coughing.
- In hospitalised patients, salbutamol and chlorpromazine may be used to supress the cough.
- Attention to feeding is essential to prevent dehydration and malnutrition.
- Physiotherapy may help prevent or improve pulmonary complications.
- Rectal prolapse is treated by manual reduction and strapping of the buttocks with Elastoplast®.

Prevention
- Routine immunisation is essential. Only children with a history of convulsions are not immunised against pertussis.
- Prevent contact between small babies and children who have pertussis wherever possible.
- Pertussis vaccine is not given after two years of age.
- Children who are household contacts should receive a course of erythromycin.

HIV infection

Definition

The Human Immunodeficiency Virus (HIV) is the cause of the Acquired Immune Deficiency Syndrome (AIDS). In an infected child, the virus invades and later destroys the CD4 lymphocytes and other immune-related cells whose numbers are reduced. This results in suppression of immunity, which leads to frequent and severe infections, poor growth, chronic diarrhoea, and a shortened lifespan.

Children acquire the virus in a number of ways. The most common is by mother-to-child transmission (MTCT). The baby is most commonly infected with the virus during labour and vaginal delivery and to a lesser extent during pregnancy and breastfeeding. The risk of transmission is 5% during pregnancy, 15% during a vaginal delivery, and 15% during two years of mixed breastfeeding if antiretroviral prophylaxis or therapy is not used. Children can also be infected by sexual abuse and, in rare cases, by blood transfusion.

It is important to understand that not all children are affected by the virus to the same degree. There are those who show rapid progress and who die early. Equally there are others who show much slower progress and who survive longer. Realising this together with the advent of antiretroviral treatment, it is important for health workers to be convinced that good medical and social management of affected children can greatly improve the quality and quantity of their lives and, therefore, is very worthwhile.

Prevention

Programmes to prevent mother-to-child transmission (PMTCT) involve giving one or preferably more antiretroviral drugs to the mother before and during labour and to the baby after delivery to prevent the virus from infecting the baby. Routine counselling and voluntary testing of mothers in early pregnancy to see if MTCT prevention is needed are a vital part of the programme. HIV transmission during pregnancy and delivery can be reduced from 20 to less than 5% with antiretroviral prophylaxis.

Because of the risk of breast milk transmission, the method of feeding infants at risk is important in prevention. A mother must be given the opportunity to make an informed choice. She should be informed and encouraged to choose either exclusive breastfeeding or exclusive formula feeding. The best way to prevent breast milk transmission of the virus is to avoid all breast milk and to feed milk formula. The next best method is to give exclusive breast milk alone with no formula, water or solids. However, the mother must be allowed to make her own choice and then be supported in her decision. The most dangerous regimen is to feed both breast milk and formula (mixed feeding). In a poor household it may be best to advise exclusive breastfeeding for six months rather than exclusive (expensive) formula feeding. The health professional's role is to counsel and advise on the best method of feeding an HIV exposed newborn on an individual basis, depending on the individual's circumstances.

Clinical progress
On entering the infant, the virus reproduces rapidly in the immune system. After a latent period lasting from a few months up to several years, during which time the child is apparently well, the number of virus particles increases. As this happens, the child's immunity is increasingly damaged and the telltale signs and symptoms of clinical AIDS appear.

The clinical severity of HIV infection in children is graded from stage 1 to 4. Children with stage 4 are said to have AIDS.

Reasons to suspect that a child might be HIV positive or even have symptomatic HIV infection
- The mother is known to be HIV positive.
- Some of the typical symptoms and signs are present.
- Exposure to sexual abuse.

Common symptoms and signs of HIV infection in a child:
- Poor or unsatisfactory weight gain or weight loss.
- Diarrhoea – either frequent episodes or chronic.
- Frequent sore mouth due to thrush.
- Difficulty swallowing from extensive thrush.
- Frequent and severe respiratory infections or the development of TB.
- Severe nappy rash.
- Ear discharge.
- Generalised lymph node enlargement.
- Enlarged liver and / or spleen.
- Seborroeic eczema – nappy area, neck fold, and scalp.
- Chronic itchy papular skin rash.
- Chronic parotid gland enlargement.

Diagnosis

The diagnosis of HIV infection is made by carrying out antibody tests on a baby or child in whom there is reason to suspect exposure to HIV.

On suspicion of the diagnosis, the mother or guardian is counselled and, if permission is obtained, the ELISA test is done. If a baby under 18 months is tested positive, a PCR test is then done.

- ELISA: This is the most common and cheapest test but it can give a false positive result in children up to 18 months of age. This is due to the mother's HIV antibody crossing the placenta during pregnancy. After 18 months of age, a positive ELISA test is diagnostic of HIV infection.
- PCR: This test is specific for the virus and indicates definite HIV infection in the child if it is positive at any age. It is more expensive than the ELISA and often is not done routinely. It is very useful in infants under 18 months to decide whether they are HIV infected or only HIV exposed. In an infant who has never been breastfed it can be done at six weeks of age.

Often the mother discovers her own infection once her child is diagnosed and she needs to be counselled for this.

Complications of HIV infection in children
- TB: This is common and must be constantly looked for.
- Pneumocystis pneumonia: This is a very severe and life-threatening acute pneumonia with marked tachypnoea and severe cyanosis. It usually requires advanced care in hospital.
- Chronic lung disease with chronic cough, finger clubbing, and tachypnoea is common. It is often difficult to differentiate from TB.
- Chronic otorrhoea.
- Severe thrush involving the pharynx and oesophagus, which makes swallowing difficult.
- A chronic papular itchy skin rash that looks somewhat like scabies.
- Developmental delay due to involvement of the central nervous system.

The medical management of an HIV positive baby / child
This is a multifaceted process. It is helpful for the mother / caretaker and the child to attend a clinic monthly to ensure that they are getting good medical management. The activities of such a clinic include:

Growth monitoring

This is important in order to ensure good nutrition and to detect problems such as TB at an early stage.

Nutrition

HIV infected children have greater than normal nutritional requirements. It is thus important to ensure good feeding using the available feeding schemes if necessary.

Immunisation

HIV positive children need routine immunisations as much if not more than HIV negative children. They need to get their immunisations at the normal times with the exception of children with clinical signs of AIDS who should not receive BCG.

Micronutrients and vitamin supplements

It has been found that supplementing a number of micronutrients in HIV positive children improves their general health and resistance to infection:

- Zinc: Elemental zinc 5 ml daily.
- Iron: Elemental iron 1 mg/kg daily.
- Folic acid: 2,5 mg daily.
- Vitamin A:
  - Non breastfed infants 0–5months: A single oral dose of 50 000 IU at six weeks.
  - All infants 6–11 months: A single oral dose of 100 000 IU at age six months or up to 11 months.
  - All children 12–60 months: A single oral dose of 200 000 IU at 12 months, then repeated every six months until 60 months.
  - Record on Road to Health Card.
  - Do not give vitamin A to a child who has had a dose less than a month before.
  - Multivitamin treatment is not a contraindication for vitamin A.
- Multivitamins.
- Deworming: Six-monthly

Preventing of Pneumocystis pneumonia

Co-trimoxazole three times a week in the following doses:

- 5 ml if under 5 kg
- 7,5 ml if 5–10 kg
- 10 ml if 11 –15 kg, and
- 15 ml if over 15 kg.

Alternatively, a single dose daily for five days a week like the TB DOTS.
• Six weeks to two months: (2,5 to 5 kg) 2,5 ml.
• 2–12 months: (5–10 kg) 5 ml.
• 12–24 months: (10–15 kg) 7,5 ml.

Early management of infections
Treatment of infections needs to be done early and thoroughly including referral for hospital admission when necessary.

Continuity of care
As this is a chronic disorder, it is helpful if the mother / guardian and the child can build up a relationship with a clinical team who will look after them at all stages of the problem including antiretroviral therapy. Clinical supervision should be as convenient to the mother and child as possible and local facilities are desirable.

Antiretroviral therapy
When the immunological severity (low CD4 count) and clinical staging (3 or 4) of the HIV infection reaches a certain level, antiretroviral therapy is indicated. The aim is to suppress the number of viral particles in the system, allowing CD4 lymphocytes to build up and maintain immune activity at a near normal level. This will greatly improve the child's quality of life and life expectancy. Before treatment is started, the level of immune suppression is measured by means of the CD4 count and the number of viral particles in the blood is measured by means of the HIV viral load count. These two tests are also used to monitor the progress of treatment. Education and treatment readiness of the caregiver, a commitment to good adherence of the dosing schedule, and family support are essential for successful treatment. Antiretroviral treatment is best started at a special HIV clinic.

Common regimens at present include three of the following drugs:
• Zidovudine – AZT®.
• Lamivudine – 3TC®.
• Stavudine – d4T®.
• Efavirenz®.
• Kaletra®.

Detailed national regimens of first- and second-line combinations of antiretroviral drugs are available. Antiretroviral treatment should be started at a special HIV clinic. Treatment is only started if the mother or caretaker has been fully informed and is 'treatment ready'.

The HIV virus develops resistance to any one of the antiretroviral (ARV) drugs alone very quickly. In order to prevent this, at least three of the drugs are used together (multi-drug therapy). Mothers / caretakers are encouraged to complete tick sheets for the administration of each dose of medication. This ensures strict adherence to the treatment regimen which is essential to prevent the development of resistance. At the follow-up clinic the tick sheets as well as old pill packets and medicine bottles are examined, leftover medicine measured, and the adherence to the regimen regularly assessed. The ARV programme is a lifelong one and the mother / caretaker and the whole family need to become involved and be supported as they carry the burden of ensuring absolutely regular medication.

On effective treatment, the children have good appetites, gain weight, and have fewer episodes of infection.

The social issues affecting children living with AIDS

Mother's physical health

In almost all cases the mother is HIV positive and needs medical supervision and, at some stage, ARV therapy. The mother needs to be as healthy as possible to care for the child. If possible, clinics should cater for mothers and children at the same time and place.

Mother's and caretaker's emotional needs

Looking after a child with HIV/AIDS is very demanding. It is made worse emotionally by feelings of guilt and inadequacy. The health and social welfare professionals need to provide as much non-threatening support and help as possible.

Disclosure to the family

It is very difficult for a mother to get the help and support she needs to care for an HIV affected child if she does not disclose the nature of the illness to the key members of the family and / or household. She needs to be supported and encouraged to make the disclosure as early as possible.

Child care

Many children have lost one or both parents from AIDS. In this case, they will usually live with grandparents or other relatives but in some cases they need welfare assistance with formal foster or residential care. Children not living with parents or grandparents are particularly vulnerable to sexual or other abuse.

Household income

This is often limited by illness in the family. The household also experiences extra expenses in the need for regular clinic / hospital attendances. In South Africa, the child support grant should be applied for. In addition, a child with AIDS is also entitled to the Care Dependency Grant.

Chapter 12

Ophthalmology

Blepharitis
Definition
Inflammation of the eyelid margins.

Cause
• Usually bacterial, for example Staphylococcus.
• May be allergic.

Clinical features
• Crusting and scaling; the lids become glued together.
• Burning and itching of lids.

Management
• Daily cleaning of lids with moist cotton wool.
• Appropriate antibiotic eye ointment, for example chloramphenicol.
• May require special anti-allergic drops or ointment. Refer to an eye clinic if persistent and severe.

Cataract
Definition
Opacity of the lens.

Types
• Congenital cataracts, for example after maternal rubella.
• Hereditary (familial).
• Degenerative cataract, for example diabetes, trauma to lens or long-term steroid treatment.

Clinical features
• Progressive painless loss of vision.
• Grey or white opacity seen in pupil.
• Grey or white opacities in the lens seen when shining a light into eye.
• Loss of the red reflex.

Management
- Refer for correct diagnosis and further treatment.
- Any child of any age with even the suspicion of a cataract must be referred for assessment.
- Prevention where possible.

Acute conjunctivitis

Definition
A common acute disorder with conjunctival inflammation that can be caused by viruses, allergy or bacterial infection.

Clinical features
It is important to take a detailed history, especially when considering allergy as a cause.

Infectious
- Bacterial, for example Staphylococcus, Pneumococcus, and Haemophilus:
  - Purulent discharge with lid swelling; eyelids sticky in the morning.
  - Not itchy.
- Viral, for example Adenovirus:
  - Clear discharge with minimal swelling.
  - Not itchy.

Management of infectious conjunctivitis
- Bacterial infections: Antibiotic eye drops, for example chloramphenicol into both eyes.
- If no response to antibiotics after two or three days, refer as there may be a resistant organism.
- If only one eye is infected, prevent infection from spreading to the other eye.

Allergic
- Clear, mucoid discharge.
- Severe swelling.
- Very itchy.
- Commonly seasonal or related to a particular allergen, for example grass pollen.

Management of allergic conjunctivitis

- Mild cases may be managed with antihistamine eye drops (e.g. Spersallerg®) but if more severe, add oral antihistamine such as Phenergan® or chlorpheniramine.
- Referral: No improvement on treatment.

Foreign body

- Trauma of the eye requires careful examination to determine the extent of injury and the presence of foreign material.
- All patients with a foreign body in the eye or penetrating wounds of eye must be referred immediately.

Hyphema (Traumatic)

Definition

Bleeding into the anterior chamber following blunt injury.

Clinical features

- Eye usually red and painful.
- Blood level in anterior chamber.
- Partial or complete loss of vision if bleeding is severe.

Management

- Bed rest.
- Sedation.
- Eye pads.
- Refer if any visual impairment.

Meibomian cyst

Small firm swelling within a meibomian gland on the eyelid. Caused by a blockage of the gland duct with sebaceous material. The cyst becomes a round painless projection on the conjunctival surface of the lid. Repeated secondary infection common, causing pain and swelling.

Management

- May discharge contents and subside spontaneously.
- Refer for incision and curettage if persists.
- If secondary infection, give local antibiotic ointment. Refer when settled or if no improvement.

Phlyctenular conjunctivitis

See Infectious diseases, p. 233.

Stye (Hordeolum)

Definition
Infection of an eyelash follicle.

Causative organism
Staphylococcus usually responsible.

Clinical features
- Painful, red, and tender lid margin.
- Small round area of induration develops.
- Abscess ruptures with discharge of pus and relief of pain.

Management
- Removal of the lash at point of induration.
- Warm water bathing of eye hastens drainage.
- Antibiotic ophthalmic solution or ointment, for example chloramphenicol.
- Incision (rarely necessary).

Squint

Definition
A squint is a disorder where both eyes do not gaze exactly in the same direction. The underlying problem is in the external eye muscles. Either one or more is paralysed or, more commonly, there is uncoordinated action of the external eye muscles.

Causes
- There is strong familial tendency to squint.
- A central nervous system disease causing damage to the nerves to one or more eye muscles, for example brain tumour.
- An abnormality in the eye itself, for example cataract or tumour.

All children with suspected or obvious squint should be referred immediately for ophthalmological opinion. If a parent says a child squints, assume the squint is present until disproved by an ophthalmologist.

Examining for squint
- Hold a light source about one metre from patient and observe light reflected on cornea. If light reflections are over corresponding points of the pupils, no squint is present. If reflections are asymmetrical, proceed to next test.

- Hold light source about one metre from patient and cover one eye. If the remaining uncovered eye moves to take up fixation on the light, an obvious squint is present.
- Repeat on the other eye. Again using a light source one metre from patient, cover the eyes alternately. If there is movement of each eye to take up fixation on the light, a latent squint is present.

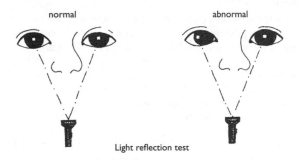

Light reflection test

Figure 12.1 Examination for squint

Wide epicanthic folds may give a false impression of a squint. Pinching the bridge of the nose of such a patient so as to reduce its width helps to determine whether or not a squint is present.

Children do not grow out of squints. After the age of six years, blindness in one eye may occur (central suppression of one image); therefore, early detection, referral, and treatment are essential.

Excessive tearing
Definition
Excessive tears from an eye in a newborn or very young infant due to narrowing of the naso-lachrymal duct.

Clinical features
Begins between three and 12 weeks of age. Tearing from the affected eye is seen. The blocked tears in the naso-lachrymal sac usually become infected and pus is seen in the eye.

Management
- Pressure on the nasolacrimal sac and gentle massage usually clears the duct of mucus plugs.

- Refer if tearing continues for more than two weeks, as prolonged blockage can lead to infection of the lacrimal sac.
- Probing by an eye specialist can be successfully performed if massage not sufficient.

Trachoma

Definition
Chronic infective keratoconjunctivitis caused by a Chlamydia organism. It is endemic in poverty-stricken areas, and associated with crowded and unsanitary living conditions. It is a leading cause of blindness.

Clinical features
- Thickening of conjunctiva with translucent follicles.
- Cornea invaded by new blood vessels.
- Eventually corneal scarring.

The cornea may be damaged by entropion (lid margin turned inward) with trichiasis (lashes that turn inwards against the cornea).

Management
- Prevention and education.
- Improved living conditions and personal hygiene.
- Tetracycline eye ointment to treat Chlamydia infection.
- Surgical correction of scarring.

Chapter 13

Parasites

Parasitic infection is very common (up to 100% of children in certain geographical areas).

Concentrate on those parasitic infections common in your area. Such parasitic infections are often obscure, or change, or hide other underlying pathology, so be careful of attributing all signs or symptoms to common parasitic infections in an endemic area, and remain aware of the possibility of dual pathology.

Amoebiases
An infestation with *Entamoeba histolytica* (Protozoal organism).

Epidemiology
- Worldwide – all age groups.
- Soil conditions.
- Hygiene.

Clinical features
- Often symptomless.
- Abdominal complaints of flatulence, diarrhoea, abdominal discomfort.
- Dysentery (blood and mucus) – mild or severe.

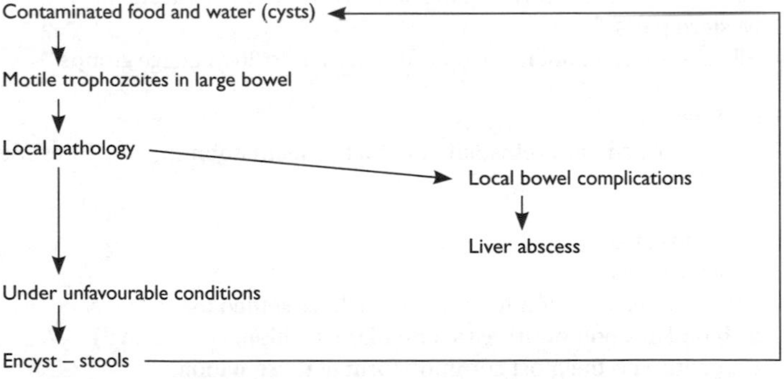

Contaminated food and water (cysts)

Motile trophozoites in large bowel

Local pathology

Local bowel complications

Liver abscess

Under unfavourable conditions

Encyst – stools

Figure 13.1 Life cycle of *Entamoeba hystolytica*: faecal ⟶ oral

- Local complications:
  - Peritonitis from perforation of bowel.
  - Amoeboma (mass in bowel).
  - Intestinal haemorrhage.
  - Ongoing colitis.
- Liver abscess:
  - Tender, enlarged liver and high fever.

Diagnosis
- Suspect it in all cases of diarrhoea with blood and mucus.
- Refer to hospital for:
  - Microscopy of warm stool for amoebae and / or cysts.
  - Proctoscopy / sigmoidoscopy – ulcer scrapings for microscopy.

Treatment
- Metronidazole (Flagyl®) suspension 200 mg/5 ml, three to four times daily for five days.
- Treat diarrhoea, fluid loss, etc.
- Local complications: May require surgery, liver abscess drainage or bowel perforation closure / resection.
- Prevention: Water supply, sanitation, washing food.

Bilharzia (Schistosomiasis)
Infestation with *Schistosoma haematobium* or *S. mansoni*.

Epidemiology
- Found in many countries. Extensive in South Africa, except for south-western parts.
- All ages affected, but more common in ten- to 20-year age groups.

Pathology
Eggs deposited in veins of bladder (haematobium) or intestine (mansoni).

Clinical features
- Fever, skin rash.
- Liver enlarged and tender after larvae have settled there. Followed by blood in stools or urine (at end of micturition, i.e. terminal). Haematuria is the most common form of presentation.

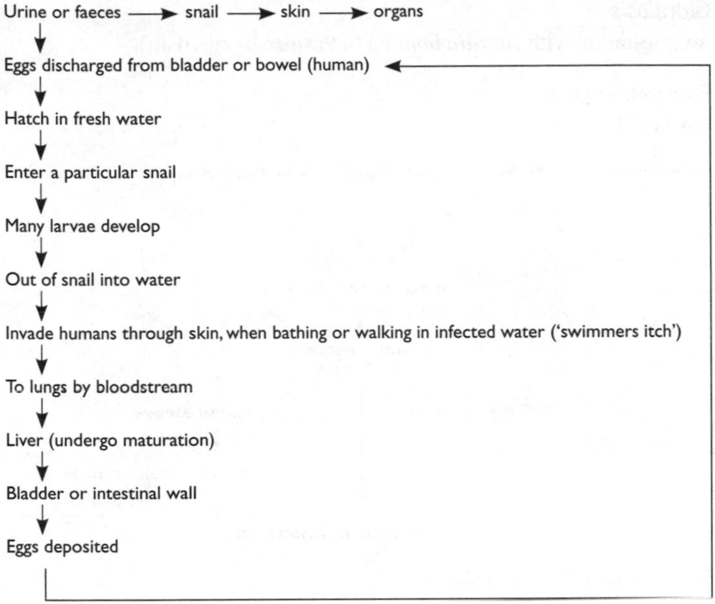

Urine or faeces ⟶ snail ⟶ skin ⟶ organs
↓
Eggs discharged from bladder or bowel (human) ◄─────────────────┐
↓   │
Hatch in fresh water   │
↓   │
Enter a particular snail   │
↓   │
Many larvae develop   │
↓   │
Out of snail into water   │
↓   │
Invade humans through skin, when bathing or walking in infected water ('swimmers itch')
↓   │
To lungs by bloodstream   │
↓   │
Liver (undergo maturation)   │
↓   │
Bladder or intestinal wall   │
↓   │
Eggs deposited ───┘

Figure 13.2 Life cycle of Bilharzia

Diagnosis
Finding eggs in urine (haematobium – spine at end) or in stool (mansoni – lateral spine).

Treatment
Refer for accurate diagnosis and treatment with:
- Biltricide® (Praziquantel).
- Bilarcil® (Oxamniquine).
- Ambilhar® (Niridazole).

Prevention
- Control snails in water (public health measures).
- Do not bathe or walk in infected water.
- Sanitation: Avoid using rivers or riverbanks as toilets.

Giardiasis

An infestation with *Giardia lamblia* (a Protozoal organism).

Epidemiology

Worldwide.

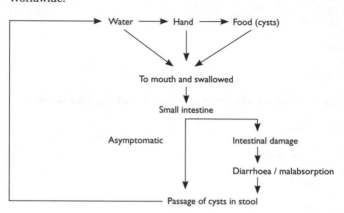

Figure 13.3 Life cycle of Giardia

Clinical features

- Very often symptomless.
- Explosive, watery, foul diarrhoea with abdominal distension.
- Fever, gaseous production with belching and flatus.
- Chronic / subacute (or intermittent) diarrhoea.
- Often a problem in crèches.

Complications

- Failure to thrive due to malabsorption from intestinal mucosal damage.
- Complications of acute diarrhoea.
- Asymptomatic cyst carriers infecting others.

Diagnosis

Requires referral for carrying out of stool examination, duodenal intubation and aspiration, or duodenal biopsy.

Treatment

- Metronidazole (Flagyl® suspension):
  - Under 15 kg: 500 mg.
  - 15–22 kg: 800 mg.
  - Over 22 kg: 1 gram daily for five days.
- In most cases, giardiasis is treated on clinical suspicion alone.

Prevention

Boil water for ten minutes before drinking if there is any doubt about safety of water supply.

Hookworm

An infestation with *Ancylostoma duodenale* or *Necator americanus*.
A very common parasite in tropical countries.

Epidemiology

Twenty-five per cent of population in tropical countries infected.

Clinical features

- 'Ground itch' of skin (larval entry site).
- Abdominal pain.
- Iron deficiency anaemia (may be severe), as parasite is a blood sucker.

Complications

- Severe anaemia.
- Cardiac failure (secondary to severe anaemia).

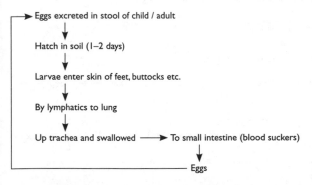

Figure 13.4 Life cycle of Hookworm: Faecal ⟶ skin

- Failure to thrive.
- Hypoalbuminaemia.

Diagnosis
Eggs in stool.

Treatment
- Mebendazole: 500 mg single dose for children over two years.
or
- Albendazole:
  - Children between 1 and 2 years: 200 mg single dose.
  - Children over 2 years: 400 mg single dose.

Prevention
- Sanitation: To avoid eggs in stools contaminating soil.
- Public health measures.

Hydatid disease
An infestation with *Echinococcus granulosa* (dog tape worm).
The adult worm is the small dog tapeworm. Normal life cycle is between dog and sheep.

Child ingests eggs via contamination with dog faeces (i.e. is now 'the sheep')

↓

Embryos penetrate duodenal wall

↓

Infest liver (usually), or lungs, brain, bone or any other organ

↓

Cyst formation (containing daughter cysts)

↓

Compression of organ or surrounding tissue

Figure 13.5 Life cycle of Hydatid tape worm: Usually dog ⟶ sheep ⟶ dog, etc.

Epidemiology
Worldwide. More common in sheep- and cattle-raising countries or areas.

Symptoms
These are due to local compression, infection, mass, etc.

Treatment
Surgical removal of the cyst is usually the only cure.
If inoperable: Albendazole10 mg/kg given twice daily for 28 days may be effective.

Pinworm
Infestation with *Enterobius vermicularis*.
The adult female worm is up to 3,5 mm (1/3 inch) long.

Epidemiology
Worldwide. Especially common where children sleep in overcrowded conditions.

Infective ova are ingested from fingers, soiled night clothes, etc.
↓
Larvae hatch out in duodenum.
↓
Larvae migrate to caecum and attach themselves to mucosa where they mature.
↓
Females laden with ova migrate out of the anus at night and deposit several thousand eggs. This causes severe itching and scratching (pruritus ani and vaginitis).
↓
Child scratches anus, and fingers pick up ova.

Figure 13.6 Life cycle of Pinworm: Faecal ⟶ oral

Note: Ova become infective a few hours after being deposited.

Clinical features
- Perianal itching and scratching at night.
- Insomnia or restless sleeper from itching.
- Often no symptoms.

Common complications
- Trauma and secondary infection of perianal areas involved in scratching.
- Appendicitis.
- Vaginitis.

Diagnosis
- Inspection (by parent, if necessary) of perianal area at night when itching is intense. Active female worms are often seen.
- Recovery and microscopic identification of ova from perianal skin. Apply sticky tape to anus at night. In morning detach, stick tape onto microscope slide, and examine under microscope for ova.
- Worm ova not often seen in stools.

Treatment
- Mebendazole: 500 mg single dose for children over two years.
or
- Albendazole:
  - Children between one and two years: 200 mg single dose.
  - Children over two years: 400 mg single dose.
- Repeat after two weeks.

Advice to parents
- Explain nature of condition.
- Bath regularly.
- Avoid scratching.
- Cut nails short.

Pneumocystis pneumonia
Infection by *Pneumocystis jiroveci* (a fungal organism) in an immuno-compromised child or HIV patient; see Chapter 11 on HIV (pp. 243–249).
Worldwide distribution: Pets / rodents / human carriers.

Diagnosis
- Chest X-ray.
- Bronchial brushing / lavageor lung biopsy.

Treatment
Co-trimoxazole (Septran® / Bactrim®): 5 mg/kg/dose (trimethoprim component) (maximum 300 mg) six-hourly intravenously.

Roundworm
Infestation with *Ascaris lumbricoides*.
Adult worms are 10–20 cm long, and look like garden earthworms.

Epidemiology
Occurs in moist warm climates. It is very common in children aged one to five years in Cape Town – the crawling, 'dirt playing' ages.

Child ingests infective ova with dirt or soil. ◄─────────────┐

↓

Ova hatch in duodenum to become larvae, which cross gut wall into blood vessels and eventually reach lungs.

↓

Larvae leave pulmonary capillaries and enter alveolar air spaces, then move up trachea and are swallowed where larvae mature and live in small intestine.

↓

Many ova (about 200 000 per day, per female worm) are passed in child's faeces and the cycle of infection continues. ───────────────────────────────┘

Figure 13.7 Life cycle of Roundworm (lives for 1–2 years): Faecal ⟶ oral

Note: Ova need about two weeks outside the body to become infective.

Clinical features
- The most common sign is the passage of worms from the anus. Sometimes they are vomited or come out through mouth or nose, especially if child is pyrexial.
- There may be low grade fever and listlessness.
- Abdominal colic may occur.
- High fever or other gastrointestinal disturbances in the child may result in increased passage of worms (vomited up or passed rectally).
- There may be no symptoms in some cases.
- Roundworms may affect nutrition in malnourished children.

Diagnosis
History of passing worms, or finding these or their ova in stool.

Common complications
- Worms in common bile duct may give rise to severe upper abdominal pain and vomiting. Jaundice is rare.
- Small bowel obstruction by mass of worms.
- Migration from capillaries into the alveolae of lungs may precipitate bronchospasm in susceptible individuals.
- May have an 'allergic' eosinophilic response in lungs which looks like patchy consolidation on CXR.

Treatment
- Mebendazole: 500 mg single dose for children over two years.
or

- Albendazole:
  - Children between one and two years: 200 mg single dose.
  - Children over two years: 400 mg single dose.
- At primary health care facilities, routine deworming medication is given six-monthly and charted on the Road to Health Card.

Advice to parents
- Wash vegetables.
- Child to wash hands before eating.
- Avoid dirt eating (pica).
- Good faecal disposal (if no flush toilet).
- Treat all children at risk in household (under five years).

Referral
If signs suggest an acute abdomen.

Tapeworm
Infestation with *Taenia saginata* (in beef) or *Taenia solium* (in pork).

Adult:
- Small head with suckers. *T. Solium* also has hooklets.
- Body in segments, may total five metres in length.
- Adult worm may live for over ten years.

Meat ──▶ bowel ──▶ cattle / pigs ──▶ humans
│
▼
Cysticerci (larvae) ingested by humans (final host) in poorly cooked meat ◀──
│
▼
Small intestine, where head attaches itself to the mucosa
│
▼
Body grows, producing many segments (proglottids), which contain eggs
│
▼
Segments are passed in stools to ground vegetation
│
▼
Eaten by and infect cattle and / or pigs (intermediate host) and go *via* intestine to reach bloodstream
│
▼
Settles out in muscles of animal which is later eaten by humans and the cycle continues ──

Figure 13.8 Life cycle of tapeworms

Epidemiology
Widespread, especially where poorly cooked meat is eaten.

Clinical features
General:
- Passage of segments in stools.
- Malaise, anorexia, abdominal pain, distention, diarrhoea, poor growth.
- Fever, possibly due to toxic metabolic products from the worm.
- There may be no symptoms or signs.

Complications
- On ingestion of eggs of *Taenia solium,* larvae enter bloodstream and involve brain (may cause epilepsy), eye or muscles, etc. (cysticercosis). As larvae die, so calcification tends to occur with evidence on X-ray of skull and muscle or CT / MRI scan of brain. Larvae which die in the brain produce swelling around them which, in turn, may cause raised intracranial pressure (with heavy infestations) and cerebral oedema.
- Appendicitis.

Diagnosis
By finding white segments (proglottids) in stool.

Treatment
- Mebendazole: 500 mg single dose for children over two years.
- Albendazole:
  ○ Children between one and two years: 200 mg single dose.
  ○ Children over two years: 400 mg single dose.
- Specific treatment for cerebral cysticercosis:
  ○ Praziquantel is used with steroids to prevent cerebral oedema.

Prevention
- Proper inspection of meat for 'cysts' in beef and pork (termed 'measly' meat).
- Adequate cooking of meat.

Threadworm
Infestation with *Strongyloides stercoralis.*

Epidemiology
Found in tropical and sub-tropical countries.

Infected from contaminated soil (free living form) ◄──────────────┐

↓

Filariform larva penetrate skin

↓

To lungs *via* bloodstream or lymphatics

↓

Swallowed to intestine (migration up trachea)

↓

Develops in small intestine

↓

Eggs in faeces (hatch after two days) ──────────────────────────┘

Figure 13.9 Life cycle of Threadworm: Faecal ──► skin

Symptoms
- Mild (asymptomatic) to severe.
- Skin itch or eruption.
- Cough, bronchitis.
- Epigastric pain / duodenitis.
- Diarrhoea leading to malabsorption.
- Cholecystitis.

Diagnosis
Eggs in stool or larvae in duodenal aspirate.

Treatment
- Mebendazole (Vermox®): One tablet twice daily or 5 ml twice daily for three days.
- Albendazole (if older than two years): Two tablets (400 mg total) as single dose.

Prevention
- Sanitation (soil contamination).
- Public health measures.
- Wear shoes. Avoid shady areas / damp soil.

Whipworm
Infestation with *Trichuris trichiura*.
Adult worms are about 30–45 mm long. Very slender anteriorly and

stubby posteriorly. Live attached to mucosa of large bowel, where they cause blood loss from site of attachment.

Epidemiology
• Warm humid climates.
• Prevalent in southern Africa.
• Most common ages: Five to 14 months.
• Many children have light, symptomless infestations.
• Malnourished children tend to develop very heavy infestations.

Infective ova are ingested with dirt ◄─────────────────────────┐
    ▼   │
Ova hatch in duodenum   │
    ▼   │
Larvae migrate to large bowel and attach to the mucosa, where they mature and later produce adult worms in large bowel   │
    ▼   │
Ova are passed in faeces ─────────────────────────────────────┘

Figure 13.10 Life cycle of Whipworm (a lifespan of about two years): Faecal ⟶ oral

Note: Ova need about ten to 20 days in a moist soil to become infective. Typical tea-tray ova.

Clinical features
• Light worm loads: No symptoms.
• Heavy loads (1 000 or more worms):
  ○ There may be diarrhoea with blood, and rectal prolapse may occur.
  ○ Iron-deficiency anaemia may be the presenting feature and this may be severe. It is due to blood being sucked by large numbers of adult worms, and lost from mucous membrane of bowel at their sites of attachment. In a case of unexplained iron deficiency anaemia, consider the possibility of Trichuris infestation; also if iron-deficiency anaemia does not respond to treatment or recurs after adequate treatment.

Diagnosis
Definitive diagnosis is identification of typical ova by microscopy of a stool smear.

Prevention
As for Ascaris.

Treatment
- Mebendazole (Vermox®): One tablet twice daily for three days or 5 ml twice daily for three days.
- Albendazole (if older than two years): Two tablets (total 400 mg) as single dose.
- Promote good nutrition.

Advice to parents
- Explain the nature of the condition.
- Avoid infestation by:
  ○ Washing hands before eating.
  ○ Washing vegetables.
  ○ Good hygienic faecal disposal.
  ○ Preventing dirt eating.
- Improve diet; this will reduce the worm load.

Preparing a stool slide for microscopy
1. Mix stool well.
2. Place two small quantities of stool on a glass slide.
3. Add a drop or two of normal saline to one specimen and a drop or two of diluted tincture of iodine to the other.
4. Cover each specimen with a coverslip.
5. Examine under microscope for ova.

Note: If amoebae are being looked for, stool and slide must be kept warm.

Chapter 14

Renal

Common important findings

Haematuria

Definition

Passing blood in urine. This may be obvious to the naked eye (macroscopic) when the urine is dark or red, or the blood may only be found on testing with a reagent strip (microscopic).

Main causes

From the kidney:
- Acute glomerulonephritis.
- Pyelonephritis.
- Bleeding disorders.
- Kidney tumours, for example Wilm's tumour.
- Kidney tuberculosis.
- Kidney stones.

From the bladder:
- Cystitis.
- Bilharzia.

From urethra:
- Trauma.
- Infection.

Usually the brighter the blood, the lower the site of the lesion in the urinary tract.

Note: Dyes from certain foods, sweets, and drugs can cause urine to be red (as well as other colours). Test with a reagent strip (dipstick) to see if the red colour is due to blood.

Management

All cases of haematuria should be referred to hospital for investigation.

Oedema

Oedema – swelling due to fluid collecting in the tissues – is a common presenting sign in childhood. The cause can usually be determined clinically so it is important to take a detailed history. The two most common causes of oedema are nutritional and renal.

Causes

Nutritional

Kwashiorkor and marasmic kwashiorkor. Clinically there will usually be a low weight for age and other signs including skin lesions and hair changes, misery, anorexia, and apathy. It is possible that kwashiorkor can occur in a child who falls within the normal percentiles.

Renal

Nephritis and nephrotic syndrome. Clinically there may be nothing to find apart from the oedema. There may be a history of a recent sore throat, or passage of dark urine (acute nephritis). Diagnosis is made on the history and by testing the urine for protein and red cells.

Cardiac

Heart failure. In addition to the oedema there might be breathlessness, tachycardia, an enlarged liver, and distended neck veins. In small children, the early signs of heart failure are a large liver and facial oedema and there is not necessarily oedema of the feet. Check haemoglobin level and take a chest X-ray.

Hepatic

Chronic liver disease is a relatively uncommon cause of oedema in children. Look for other signs of liver damage, such as a large or firm liver, jaundice, ascites, bleeding or anaemia. Check liver function tests and serum albumin.

Allergic

Sensitivity to certain foods, beestings, insect bites, and some intestinal worms may give periorbital oedema, and sometimes a patchy oedema over the rest of the body. An urticarial rash is often present. Examine stool for parasites and check on recently introduced items of diet.

Local

Signs of sepsis, trauma, bites or stings in the area of swelling, or obstruction to blood or lymph drainage from that area.

Proteinuria

Protein in the urine when detected by testing with reagent strips suggests the possibility of kidney disease. If proteinuria persists over a period of some weeks, refer for further investigation.

Acute post-streptococcal glomerulonephritis

Definition

A condition in which swelling of the face and lower legs is accompanied by bloodstained urine and in which recovery is complete in over 95% of the cases.

Cause

This is a reaction of the kidney to a streptococcal infection of the throat or skin several weeks previously.

Pathology

There is inflammation in the glomeruli of the kidney, which results in the following:

- A reduction in the fluid filtered by kidney, which leads to reduced urine output and consequently oedema.
- Glomerular damage which shows as the passing of blood and protein in the urine.
- Unusually high reabsorption of sodium into the blood resulting in further increased blood volume, which further contributes to the swelling.

Epidemiology

- Age: Two to ten years. The condition is very rare under two years of age.
- Socio-economic status: Acute nephritis is much more common if the socio-economic status is low. It is associated with overcrowding and with increased incidence of skin infections and pharyngitis, tonsillitis, and otitis media. In all of these, streptococcal infection plays a major role.

History and clinical features

- Oedema, that is, puffy eyes in the morning and swollen feet at night.
- The urine is dark or smoky, and looks like coca-cola or tea; only occasionally is it bright red.
- Output of urine is less than usual.
- Loss of appetite.

Examination: Some or all of the following may be found:
- Oedema of the face and / or legs.
- Evidence of streptococcal infection; check throat, ears, and skin.
- Hypertension is common: It is important always to measure the blood pressure.
- Heart failure may be present in severe cases.
- Check urine with reagent strip for blood and protein.

Complications
- Severe hypertension.
- Cardiac failure due to increased blood volume. In this case, the chest X-ray shows an enlarged heart.
- Convulsions (due to raised blood pressure). Note that the patient may present with convulsions.
- Acute renal failure with raised urea and creatinine levels.

Clinical course
- Oedema with low urine output lasts from a few days to two to three weeks. A diuresis then occurs which lasts a few days.
- Urine may continue to look dark for up to six weeks. On testing with reagent strips, blood may be present for up to two years. The protein in the urine should clear within a month. Ultimate recovery occurs in most cases.

Management
Children who are swollen or who have dark urine should be referred to hospital. The treatment there will include:
- Daily weighing.
- Collection of all urine to measure volume.
- Fluid restriction (20 ml/kg/day + daily output) until diuresis occurs.
- Diet:Low sodium, low protein diet during acute phase; in practice, bread, jam, rice, salt-free vegetables, and fruit.
- Penicillin for ten days; local treatment of skin sepsis.
- Diuretics: One or two doses of furosemide will often help to reduce the oedema.
- Bed rest until naked eye haematuria has gone, that is, urine colour has returned to normal.

Treatment of complications
Hypertension, convulsions, cardiac failure, and acute renal failure all need specific treatment in hospital.

Prognosis

Ninety-five per cent recover completely. This may take up to two years. Second attacks are rare if recovery from the initial attack has been complete.

Nephrotic syndrome

Definition

In this condition, there is a heavy loss of protein in the urine. This results in a low serum albumin and generalised oedema.

Aetiology

In 75% of cases in childhood, the cause is unknown (idiopathic). The remaining 25% of cases occur as part of a variety of disorders such as unresolved acute nephritis, purpura, lupus, drugs, hepatitis B, and congenital syphilis.

Epidemiology

Worldwide. Very rare under one year. More common in boys under five years, but may occur at any age.

Clinical features

- Gradual onset of oedema, which presents in the face in early morning, feet later in the day.
- Abdominal swelling due to ascites may occur.
- Heavy albuminuria on reagent strips. There is usually no blood, but haematuria may occur.
- Blood pressure is normal in idiopathic cases, but may be raised in other types.

Management

Any child suspected of having nephrotic syndrome should be referred for hospital investigation and treatment. Hospital management includes:
- Normal diet.
- Diuretics / intravenous albumin.
- Steroids in certain types.

Prognosis

Idiopathic type (no haematuria):

Majority ultimately recover, but there may be many relapses; not regarded as cured until urine is protein-free for at least five years.

Other types (haematuria often present):
Prospects of full recovery not as good as idiopathic type.

Urinary tract infection
Definition
Bacterial infection of the urinary tract, which includes the kidneys, ureter, bladder, and urethra.

Pathology
E. coli and *Proteus* are the most common organisms. The organisms probably enter the bladder *via* the urethra and reach the kidneys by reflux of urine up the ureter during the passage of urine. In infants, the organism may enter *via* the bloodstream.

Conditions that predispose to infection:
- Congenital abnormalities of the urinary tract make infection much more likely, for example hydronephrosis, duplex kidney, etc.
- Kidney or bladder stones.

Epidemiology
- Common in early childhood, including the newborn period.

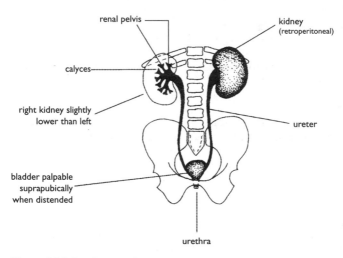

Figure 14.1 Renal system: Basic anatomy

- Under six months, incidence equal in both sexes; thereafter, females predominate four to one.

Clinical features

- In young children, features may not suggest involvement of the urinary tract. Fever rigors, vomiting, diarrhoea, abdominal pain, convulsions, poor appetite, and failure to thrive may occur and can be confused with any acute infection of infancy. Jaundice may occur in the very young infant. There must be a high index of suspicion in the sick young infant.
- Older children may complain of frequent painful passage of urine, back pain or suprapubic pain. Enuresis may appear, which is particularly important if bladder control had already been established. The other features noted in young children may also occur.

Investigation

Urine specimens should be collected and submitted for microscopy, culture, and sensitivity. This will identify the organisms and their antibiotic sensitivity.

Urine collection:
- In infants: Use a plastic collection bag after cleaning perineum with soap and water.
- In older children: Collect a clean sample from mid-stream urine flow.

Diagnosis

Infected urine contains pus cells and bacteria. These can be screened for with the urine reagent strips that have leucocyte and nitrite patches. Nitrite is a product of bacterial metabolism and is a marker for the presence of many bacteria in the urine; leucocytes are a marker for inflammation.

It is important to be certain about the diagnosis, as all children with true urinary tract infections will need further investigation. A urine sample collected by suprapubic aspiration is important in newborn infants, as bag specimens are often contaminated.

Complications

- Septicaemia in the newborn and very young infants.
- Pyelonephritis may cause permanent renal damage, especially under two years.

Management

General

- Anti-fever measures.
- Adequate fluid intake.

Specific

The recent problem with treatment of urinary tract infections is the resistance of the common organisms to many antibiotics. Obtaining a culture and sensitivity is, therefore, essential to allow correct treatment. Initially use Augmentin® or Cefuroxime for seven days. In cases of septicaemia, more powerful antibiotics may be necessary (e.g. gentamicin). Success of therapy should be checked by a repeat urine examination five days after stopping therapy.

Further investigation

All children who have had a urinary tract infection need an ultrasound examination of the renal tract, and in children under two years, a micturating cystourethrogram (MCUG) examination should be considered to exclude the presence of urinary tract abnormalities and / or reflux.

Long-term therapy

Children with significant reflux are often put on long-term anti-bacterial treatment to prevent further attacks and consequent renal scarring. They sometimes need surgery to abolish the reflux. Follow-up routine urine cultures should be done in this group.

Enuresis

Definition

This is bed-wetting at night due to the delayed acquisition of normal bladder control during sleep. It is the involuntary and consistent episodic bed-wetting during sleep by a child over the age of six years, that is, after the age by which normal bladder control would be expected.

Classification

- Usually the child has never been dry at night. This variety seldom has an organic urinary tract cause (primary enuresis).
- When wetting recurs after a period of dryness, the problem is more likely to have an underlying organic or emotional cause (secondary enuresis).

Diagnosis

This involves taking a full history, with emphasis on environmental, psychological, social, and emotional factors. Be careful about making the diagnosis if bed-wetting comes on after a long period of dryness. Then think about other causes such as urinary tract infection, diabetes mellitus or emotional causes.

Clinical examination

- Exclude abnormalities of the external genitalia.
- Exclude abdominal swelling or mass (e.g. enlarged kidneys).
- Observe the child while he or she is micturating. A poor stream in boys may indicate posterior urethral valves.

Test the urine to exclude

- Urinary tract infection.
- Diabetes mellitus.

Management

- Support, encouragement, and understanding is essential.
- Specific aspects:
  - Fluid restriction after supper.
  - Lifting the child to empty the bladder at night; the child must wake fully.
  - Reward and disappointment ('star' charts).
- Medication (this results in dryness only while medication is taken):
  - Imipramine 10–20 mg at night or Oxybutynin 5 mg twice daily for child over five years; maximum dose 5 mg three times daily.
- Follow-up.
- Reasons for referral:
  - If an underlying urinary tract abnormality is suspected.
  - Persistent enuresis.
  - Secondary enuresis without emotional factors.

Respiratory tract

Asthma and wheezing (Lower airway obstruction)

If the smaller airways (bronchi and bronchioles) are narrowed for any reason, the result will be difficulty in breathing which worsens on expiration. This is because airways in the chest are squeezed during breathing out. Air is then progressively trapped in the lungs, leading to over-inflation.

Causes of airway narrowing

- **Infection**: Airway wall oedema and mucus causing narrowing.
- **Asthma**:Usually hyper-reactive bronchial muscle reacting to many stimuli such as exercise, allergy, irritant gases, etc.
- **Foreign bodies**: These block the lumen of the airway directly.
- **External pressure**: This may be from a variety of causes, but tuberculous lymph nodes are one of the most common.

Clinical signs

- Respiratory distress.
- Wheezing.
- Over-inflation of the lungs.
- Liver and spleen pushed down into the abdomen by the flattened diaphragm.

Asthma

Definition

Usually a familial disorder in which the bronchial muscle is unusually sensitive to external stimuli and responds by constricting. This leads to repeated episodes of reversible lower airway obstruction. This presents with wheezing and cough which is relieved by a bronchodilator.

Some typical external stimuli:
- Exercise.
- Viral chest infection.
- Changes in temperature and weather.
- Allergy to inhaled or ingested allergens, for example house dust mite.

Clinical progress

The asthmatic child typically has repeated attacks of lower airway obstruction in infancy and childhood. The diagnosis is made over a period of time, after a child has had a number of episodes. Often presents with persistent night-time and early morning coughing or wheezing. May only have coughing spells without wheezing. The peak expiratory flow rate, which can be measured in children from five years of age, is lower than expected for age.

Management

Acute attack

Either
- Nebulised salbutamol (Ventolin®) solution or fenoteral (Berotec®) solution alone or plus Ipratropium (Atrovent®) solution (0,5 ml each) in 1 ml saline.

Or
- An aerosol pump (metered dose inhaler) with a spacer: Two puffs (200 µg) of salbutamol or fenoterol (Berotec®). Spacers work very well, so do not need nebulisers.
- Repeat after 30 minutes if no response. If still no response, treat as acute severe asthma. It is important to recognise when an acute attack is not responding to treatment and to proceed to the management as below. Delay in this step can be life threatening.

Acute severe asthma (Status asthmaticus)

If the acute attack does not resolve rapidly after the above measures, provide face mask oxygen and refer urgently to hospital for further management.

Treatment in hospital will usually include:
- Oxygen.
- Nebulised bronchodilators.
- Intravenous fluids.
- Steroids.

Maintenance therapy

Mild intermittent asthma (occasional episodes of coughing and wheezing only with a peak flow rate of 80% or more of expected) needs treatment of the mild acute attacks with an inhaled bronchodilator. However, more severe asthma needs maintenance therapy. The aim of maintenance therapy is to prevent acute attacks.

Mild persistent asthma (more than six episodes annually with a peak flow rate of 60–80%) requires regular inhaled steroids (e.g. beclomethasone) to prevent acute attacks.

Children with more severe persistent asthma (peak flow rate less than 60%) should be referred to an asthma clinic for assessment and management:

- Daily beclomethasone (Becotide®) inhaler.
- Daily oral bronchodilators (e.g. slow release theophylline).
- Oral steroids (prednisone) in the most severe cases.

Bronchiolitis

Bronchiolitis is due to a viral infection (especially respiratory syncitial virus) of the lower respiratory tract which affects mainly the smaller airways, causing severe lower airways obstruction. It is most common between three months and two years of age, but can occur in older or younger children. It usually follows, or is accompanied by an upper respiratory tract infection.

Clinical symptoms and signs

- There is an acute onset of coughing and tachypnoea as well as poor feeding in severe cases. Apnoea may occur in neonates.
- The temperature may be normal or raised.
- On examination: Tachypnoea, tachycardia, recession, wheezing, and air trapping is found.
- Severe cases may be cyanotic.
- Chest may be 'silent' on auscultation, with very little wheezing heard, because so little air is being moved.
- Bilateral crackles develop later.
- Chest X-ray: This shows air trapping without consolidation.

Treatment

- No specific treatment is available and the lower airway obstruction clears within three to five days, even in severe cases.
- Bronchodilators are of limited value but are usually given orally or by nebulisation.
- Special care should be given to feeding and hydration. Nasogastric tube feeds are often needed.
- Antibiotics can be given to prevent secondary infection.
- Give oxygen by face-mask to all severely distressed or cyanotic children, and refer to hospital as mechanical ventilation may be

necessary. In hospital, oxygen is administered by perspex head box. If very distressed, IV fluids are given.

- Steroids are of no help.

Bronchitis

Definition

Inflammation of the bronchi caused by viral or bacterial infection. Usually follows an upper respiratory tract infection. Lower airways obstruction may occur. Repeated 'wheezy bronchitis' is usually asthma. Severe bronchitis is often part of pneumonia.

Clinical features

- Cough which may be loose or dry. Cough may cause chest pain, but never produces blood-stained sputum.
- There may be fever.
- There may be wheezing.
- Rapid or difficult breathing and cyanosis do not occur.
- Always suspect TB if cough lasts longer than two weeks.

Management

- Oral amoxicillin for one week.
- Paracetamol for pain or fever.
- Oral bronchodilator: If wheezing.
- Refer to hospital if no improvement after a week or if signs of pneumonia develop.

Viral croup

Definition

An acute inflammatory condition of the larynx (larygotracheobronchitis) caused by a viral infection.

Clinical features

- Sudden onset of a barking cough.
- There may be associated hoarseness.
- Worse at night.
- May be recurrent.
- **May develop stridor if becomes severe.**

Management

- Croup without stridor can be managed at home.
- Antifever treatment if needed.

- Co-trimoxazole (Septran® / Bactrim®) or amoxicillin for five days.
- Careful observation for signs of worsening airways obstruction with stridor.
- Do not sedate.

Advice to parents
- Moisten air around child, using steam if possible (do not give this advice if producing steam would create a fire hazard).
- Explain nature and course of illness. Indicate need to seek further help if:
  - Develops stridor.
  - Chest sucks in (recession).
  - Feeding is difficult.
  - Child is restless and anxious.

To check these points, see child the next day or, preferably, later the same day.

Indications for referral
If any of the following are present:
- Stridor (stridor may get softer with severe obstruction).
- Recession.
- Alar flare.
- Cyanosis.
- Tachypnoea.
- Child becomes restless.

Emergency treatment
Oxygen for cyanosis, to be continued during journey to hospital.

Pneumonia
Definition
Inflammation of the alveoli and small airways of the lungs due to bacterial or viral infection.

Clinical features
- The child is obviously ill, usually with fever. Sweating and rigors may occur. Cough is common.
- Breathing is rapid, shallow, and difficult and the child may grunt. There is often recession and flaring of the nostrils on inspiration.

- There may be acute chest pain on taking a deep breath, indicating pleurisy. This may be the only feature in the older child.
- The child may become drowsy; this is a dangerous sign. Oxygen saturation may be low in room air.
- On chest examination, the characteristic signs are dullness on percussion and bronchial breathing with crackles on auscultation over the consolidated area of the lung. Often in the early stages there are no abnormal auscultatory signs.

Management
- Intramuscular penicillin (amoxicillin or co-trimoxazole).
- Paracetamol (Panado®) for fever.
- If the child is cyanosed, drowsy or has difficulty breathing, give oxygen and transfer to hospital immediately.
- In milder cases, revisit at short intervals.

Advice to parents
- Explain nature and course of illness.
- Indicate need to seek further help if:
  ○ The chest sucks in on inspiration.
  ○ There is difficulty in feeding.
  ○ There is blueness of the tongue.

Indications for referral to hospital
If any one of the following is present:
- Respiration more than 60 per minute.
- Recession.
- Flaring nostrils.
- Cyanosis, drowsiness or confusion – arrange for oxygen to be given *en route* to hospital.

Follow-up:
If the pneumonia has not cleared up after ten days of treatment, do a Mantoux test and refer to TB authorities if positive.

Sinobronchitis
Definition
After an upper respiratory tract infection, the patient develops a secondary bacterial infection of the sinuses resulting in a post-nasal drip. This causes bronchitis with a chronic cough, especially at night. Frequent 'sniffing' common in allergic patients.

Management
Co-trimoxazole (Septran®, Bactrim®). If no improvement, refer to hospital.

Stridor
Definition
A high-pitched, crowing sound produced mainly during inspiration, usually due to narrowing of the trachea or larynx. Stridor is a clinical sign and is not a diagnosis. The cause must be determined.

Causes
- By far the commonest cause of laryngotracheobronchitis (LTB) is a **viral infection**, usually in a child under three years of age. Worse at night. Usually referred to as croup by the parents.
- **Measles** causing swelling of mucous membranes of larynx (either during or more than ten days after the illness). Herpes simplex infection may be a complication.
- **Laryngeal diphtheria**. Membrane in larynx causing obstruction. A membrane may also be seen on the tonsils and, if present, is a valuable clue to the diagnosis. Usually there is a marked enlargement of the lymph nodes in the neck, and fever. The child is often not seriously ill or toxic in the earlier stages.
- Inhalation of a **foreign body**.
- **Congenital abnormalities** causing obstruction of larynx, trachea or bronchi.
- Acute **epiglottitis** due to Haemophilus infection. This is a medical emergency.

Clinical features
- If due to infection, patient will usually have a temperature.
- If sudden onset and no systemic signs, consider foreign body.
- May also be associated with hoarseness of the voice, or a croupy (brassy) cough.

Management
Serious signs are:
- Distress with either restlessness or drowsiness.
- Breathing is difficult with both inspiratory and expiratory stridor.
- Pulsus paradoxus.
- Cyanosis.

- Recession.
- A membrane seen on the tonsils.

If any of these are present, transfer urgently to hospital giving oxygen. In mild stridor, refer. If not possible and if none of the above features are present, manage as follows:

- Humidify the room with steam from boiling water, keeping this well away from patient. Take care that the patient or other children do not get scalded.
- Anti-fever treatment.
- Co-trimoxazole or amoxicillin for five days.
- Follow up daily, or more often if possible, to re-assess progress or deterioration. If condition worsens or does not improve after two days, refer to hospital.

Care in hospital may include:

- Oxygen.
- IV fluids.
- Nebulised adrenaline inhalations (2 ml 1:1000 adrenaline with 2 ml saline).
- Oral prednisone 2 mg/kg.
- Intubation.
- Tracheostomy.

This is a life-threatening condition and great care must be taken in the assessment and management.

Chapter 16

Skin diseases

Abscess
See Common surgical problems, pp. 317–318.

Acne (Vulgaris)
Definition
Often referred to as teenage pimples, acne is a chronic inflammatory process of the skin occurring mostly in adolescents. It involves the sebaceous gland and its associated hair follicle. Secretions block the sebaceous canal and cause an inflammatory response in which normal skin bacteria play a role.

Causes
It is common during adolescence when there is increased sebaceous gland activity due to increased hormonal activity. Genetic factors play a role. Acne can be made worse by stress. Diet has *not* been shown to be a cause.

Epidemiology
Acne is very common, somewhat more so in males. It may be worse in humid climates.

Clinical features
Lesions occur on forehead, face, chest, back, and upper deltoid area and include 'whiteheads', 'blackheads', papules, and / or pustules.

Complications
- Scratching, squeezing, and secondary infection.
- Long-term scarring and pitting.
- Psychological problems.

Management
- Keep skin clean but avoid vigorous scrubbing.
- Moderate exposure to sunlight.

- Keratin modifying topical preparations including benzoyl peroxide and tretinoin.
- Severe cases may need oral antibiotics including erythromycin and tetracycline.
- Even more severe cases need referral for dermatological management. Treatments include topical and oral vitamin A analogue preparations and hormonal therapy in girls.

Atopic eczema

Definition

A disorder of the skin occurring with redness, minute blisters, oozing, and crusting. It is accompanied by intense itching. The longstanding lesions are dry and scaly with thickening of the skin.

Causes

- A strong genetic predisposition; also runs in families. With one atopic parent, a child has a 60% chance of having the condition, while with two atopic parents, the chances are 80%.
- The condition may be made worse by emotional factors, heat, and sweating. Scratching and secondary infection also make the condition worse.

Epidemiology

Occurs in families. Often in association with other allergic features, such as asthma and hay fever.

Clinical features

The condition changes its distribution with age and in many cases it ceases to be a problem in later childhood.

Affected children tend to have a dry skin, which needs to be managed actively.

In infancy:

- The rash starts as an area of redness with minute blisters, oozing, and crusting. It starts on the cheeks and spreads to the trunk and limbs later. The areas particularly affected are behind the knees, in front of elbows, and wrists (flexural eczema).
- Itching is intense and is made worse by warmth. The infant is often irritable and miserable.
- Local lymphadenopathy occurs due to secondary bacterial infection.

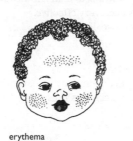

erythema
scaling
secondary infection
lymphodenopathy

Infancy

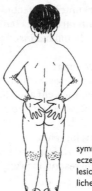

symmetrical
eczematous
lesions and
lichenification

Childhood

Figure 16.1 Distribution of atopic eczema

In later childhood:
- The lesions become chronic and the affected areas are thickened and look like leather (lichenified). Chronic scratching contributes to these changes.

Complications
Bacterial infection (usually staphylococcal or streptococcal) is very common, and is often a reason for failure of treatment.

Management
- Avoid woollen clothes.
- Perfumed soap must be avoided and be replaced with aqueous cream. Apply aqueous cream to the skin after drying.
- Moisturisation of skin using aqueous cream in the bath water.
- Manage itching with antihistamines such as Atarax® or Phenergan® given by mouth but not locally.
- Socks, gloves over hands and keep nails short to reduce scratching.
- Local ointments include: Coal tar 5% in emulsifying ointment, 1% hydrocortisone, or a steroid preparation such as Synalar® diluted 1:10 with emulsifying ointment. All are applied three times a day. The prolonged use of steroids may damage the skin, or be absorbed and retard growth.

- In recent times, the technique of wet wraps to concentrate the ointments on the affected area has been very effective.
- Clothes should be rinsed well to remove detergents.

Infected eczema:
- Use a Betadine® wash to the infected area.
- Oral erythromycin and vioform 2% in an emulsifying ointment applied locally, or Betadine® cream under an occlusive dressing.

Indications for referral:
- Severe and widespread eczema.
- Failure to respond to simple treatment after two weeks.

Note: Eczema is not a contraindication to immunisation.

Seborrhoeic dermatitis

Definition
A condition seen in normal young infants and in children with immune disorders. It is characterised by redness and scaling of the skin in a typical distribution.

Epidemiology
This is a common disorder in otherwise normal infants in whom it resolves by three to six months of age. In children with immune disorders, particularly HIV/AIDS, it either develops late or persists beyond six months and should be a cause for suspicion.

Clinical features
The condition begins with red, greasy, and scaling lesions in the scalp (cradle cap). Later it spreads to the folds of the neck, behind the ears, and the napkin area. Oozing of the skin begins later. Round, red, greasy lesions on the abdominal skin are also typical

Management
- Crusts on the scalp can be removed by applying salicylic acid 2% in Vaseline® twice a day for two days and then shampooing.
- Apply olive or vegetable oil to scalp to soften scales before shampooing to clear them.

- Selenium sulphide (Selsun®) shampooing for the scalp lesions and dilute steroid ointments applied.
- Treatment of any associated candida infection should be carried out.

Impetigo

Definition
Acute infection of superficial layers of the skin by bacteria.

Causes
Streptococci and staphylococci are the most common organisms causing infection in the epidermis of the skin. These bacteria gain entry to the skin when another problem causes damage to the epidermis as in:
- Eczema.
- Scabies.
- Insect bites.
- Head lice.

Epidemiology
- Especially common in the pre-school age group.
- More common in warm, moist climates.
- More common where hygiene is poor.
- Often spreads within households, crèches, and schools.

Clinical features
Early stage (often missed):
Non-tense blisters filled with watery pus. These very soon break down. In newborn infants, the blisters often remain intact and do not progress to crust formation.

Later stage (usually seen):
Lesions weeping and / or covered with honey-coloured crusts. These tend to heal from the centre and give a ring-like effect. Lesions may be found anywhere on the body, but especially the scalp, face, and limbs. If impetigo occurs as a complication of another skin condition, for example scabies and impetigo, the picture will be mixed.

Complications
Acute nephritis from some varieties of streptococci causing impetigo.
Pneumonia / osteitis from staphylococcal sepsis.

Management
- Hygiene: The child should be washed daily with a diluted solution of antiseptic such as Savlon®.
- Crusts must be removed after a soaking to soften them (local warm compress).
- Apply 2% vioform in zinc ointment or Betadine® ointment to affected areas three times a day until clear. This is usually about seven days.
- For scalp lesions, use Betadine® shampoo and apply 3% vioform in emulsifying ointment.
- Check scalp for lice.
- If the lesions are extensive, use an antibiotic such as erthromycin to cover staphylococcus and streptococcus.

Referral
- Lesions not improved after ten days.
- Presenting with signs of complications.

Lice
Definition
Infestation with the head louse (*Pediculosis capitis*) or pubic louse (*Pediculosis pubis*) in adolescents.

Causes
The head louse lives on the scalp where it lays its eggs which are firmly stuck to the hair shafts. The lice themselves do not cause symptoms; it is allergy to their body products which results in itching and scratching.

Epidemiology
Common, especially in school children and equally in both sexes. A whole school may be infected during group activities such as camping, etc.

Clinical features
- If no allergy has developed, there may be no symptoms.
- Itching of scalp.
- Nits (eggs) are found on the hair shaft. These are best seen in the hair just above the ears and in the nape of the neck.

Complications
Scratching leads to bacterial infection and impetigo, with localised lymph node enlargement over the back of the head and neck.

Management

- 1% gamma benzene hexachloride (lotion or shampoo): Apply to entire scalp and leave for five minutes. This kills the lice. Wash hair and comb with a nit comb. Repeat one week later.
- It may be very difficult to use a nit comb effectively in short curly hair. The scalp hair may need to be cut very short or shaved (get parents' permission for this).
- **Note:** All affected members of a household or school should be treated simultaneously.
- Treat any secondary bacterial infection as for impetigo.

Milia

Definition

A condition of newborn infants in which small white-yellow papules are found on the nose and cheeks.

Aetiology

Milia are retention cysts caused by temporary obstruction of the sebaceous gland ducts. Caused by fetal hormones.

Management

- Reassure parents that lesions will clear spontaneously over next few weeks.
- No local treatment is required.

Miliaria ('Prickly heat')

Miliaria is a common rash of infants, caused by obstruction of sweat ducts or by irritation of the skin by sweat.

Aetiology

There are two forms of miliaria. In newborn infants, the immature sweat ducts are sometimes partially obstructed. If the infant sweats excessively, sweat is trapped under the outer layer of the skin to form small vesicles. In older infants, the sweat ducts are patent but sweat may irritate the skin around the openings of the sweat ducts and thereby cause local erythema.

Clinical features

Miliaria usually occurs on the face, neck, arms, and chest. Young infants develop a rash of fine vesicles. Older infants present with a pink, macular rash (sweat rash). Both forms of miliaria are seen in infants with fever, or excessive sweating due to overheating or too many clothes.

Management
Prevention
- Keep the baby cool, especially when feverish or in hot weather.
- Avoid excessive clothing or blankets.

Treatment
- Avoid nylon clothes.
- Keep cool.
- Use baby dusting powder sparingly after washing and drying the baby carefully.
- Tepid sponge baths will decrease body heat and reverse the appearance of miliaria.

Molluscum contagiosum
Definition
Highly typical skin lesions.

Aetiology
Caused by a virus and spreads from child to child.

Epidemiology
These lesions are typically seen in children who live in large groups, for example in residential care, or in children with immune deficiency. Molluscum is an alert for HIV disease.

Clinical features
Superficial, round, about match-head size, waxy-coloured discrete lesions. They have a central depression, often with a darker spot in it (umbilicated, i.e. looks like an umbilicus).

Management
Any of the following can be tried:
- Doing nothing is best as condition will improve spontaneously.
- Prick open the roof of the lesion and shell out the contents.
- Use a light application of liquid nitrogen.
- Use a pointed orange stick dipped in phenol 1%; apply for a few seconds until lesion turns white.

Nappy rash

Definition

A dermatitis of the skin area usually covered by the baby's nappy. There are several clinical pictures, each with a different cause and treatment.

Causes

- **Ammonia**: Bacteria act on urea in the urine. This releases ammonia, which causes a chemical inflammation of the skin.
- **Monilia (thrush)**: Oral thrush is also usually present.
- **Allergy** to something in the nappy, for example detergent or fabric softener used in washing.
- **Moisture**: From delayed happy changes.

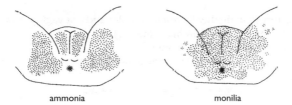

ammonia   monilia

Figure 16.2 Ammonia versus monilia nappy rash

Clinical features

- **Ammonia rash**: Red rash over area of greatest contact with the nappy. It does not penetrate into the skin creases where there is much less contact with ammonia.
- **Monilia**: Oral thrush is usually present. Small ulcers are often seen at edge of rash, which is worse in skin creases.
- **Allergy**: The rash is worse around the elastic area of waistband and leg-bands, where contact with the nappy is closest.
- **Seborrhoeic dermatitis**: An extensive red rash in the nappy area entering the folds. Usually other manifestations of seborrhoeic dermatitis elsewhere at the same time.

Management

Prevention

- Change nappies frequently.
- Apply petroleum jelly to nappy area with each nappy change (inexpensive 'brown' form is available from garages).

- Ammonia:
  - Wash the area with soap and water. Rinse and dry well.
  - Expose the buttocks to air by leaving nappies off and baby on tummy as much as possible.
  - Limit use of plastic pants.
  - Use barrier creams such as zinc oxide, for example Fissan® paste to prevent ammonia reaching skin.
  - Treat nappies by adding vinegar (a tablespoon to a ten litre bucket of water) to the final rinse. This inhibits growth of the bacteria (*Proteus*) which converts urea to ammonia.
- Monilia:
  - Treat thrush in baby's mouth, if present.
  - Expose buttocks as much as possible to air and apply Mycostatin® cream.
  - Treat thrush in mother if present (nipples and / or vagina, using cream or pessaries according to the site).
- Allergic and seborrhoea dermatitis:
  - Avoid allergens, for example change detergent or use pure soap to wash nappies.
  - Use coal tar preparation or 1% hydrocortisone.

Papular urticaria
Definition
A recurrent allergic reaction to a variety of insect bites.

Causes
Commonly due to flea or mosquito bites. The symptoms are due to an allergy to the substances injected into the skin by the insect when biting. It is a delayed hypersensitivity reaction, which recurs over years.

Epidemiology
Very common.
Fleas: These are more active in warm weather, in houses with wooden floors or carpets, and usually but NOT necessarily, cats and dogs.
Mosquitoes: Active in warm, rainy weather and where there is stagnant water.

Clinical features
- Raised itchy papules, vesicles, and bullae. Older lesions are hyperpigmented.

- Fleabites are most commonly found on the feet, lower legs, the hands and forearms of crawling infants, and in areas where the flea gets trapped against the skin by clothing such as waistbands. A row of bites in a straight line or close group is also typical (may also indicate bedbug bites).
- Mosquito bites: These are found especially on areas that are exposed at night, for example face, neck, and arms.

Complications
Bacterial infection following scratching.

Management
- Calamine lotion for itching.
- Antihistamine syrup, for example hydroxyzime (Aterax®) or trimeprazime (Vallergan®) given at night for sleep. 1% hydrocortisone in HEB for severe lesions.
- Treat any secondary infection as for impetigo.
- Mosquito repellents.
- De-flea dogs and cats in household.

Control measures for fleas:
Regular spraying with insecticide of floors, carpets, under beds and mats. Insecticide powder or flea collar for dogs and cats.

Control measures for mosquitoes:
Get rid of local stagnant water where mosquitoes breed. If control is difficult, report the problem to the local health inspector who must arrange for spraying and other control measures.

Pityriasis sicca alba
Hypo pigmented round / oval patches with diffuse borders.

Clinical features
Lesions occur mainly on the face but also on the neck, upper trunk, and arms. The lesions tend to come and go and may itch slightly.

The lesions heal spontaneously but it can take months for the pigment to return to normal. Parents can be reassured that it is not the onset of the much more serious, vitiligo. It must be differentiated from fungal infection (*Tinea vesicolor*).

Cause
The aetiology is unknown, but they are not, as commonly believed, due to worm infestation.

Treatment
No treatment necessary. Bland ointment for dryness may help.

Ringworm
Definition
Fungal infection of skin of scalp, body and / or nails.

Aetiology
Due to a variety of ringworm fungi. Note that ringworm has nothing to do with worms as is commonly believed.

Epidemiology
- *Tinea capitis* (ringworm of scalp) only occurs before puberty; the others occur at all ages.

Clinical features
- **Tinea capitis - scalp**: Circular lesions on scalp with scales and loss of hair (broken off at scalp). There are usually no symptoms. May cause a boggy granuloma with pustules.
- **Tinea corporis - body**: Round scaly patches with a clear centre and a red border which may show vesicles.
- **Tinea pedis – feet**: ('Athlete's foot') Smelly, moist peeling skin between toes.
- **Tinea vesicolor - trunk**: Pale or dark discrete to confluent areas usually on back. Slightly scaly.

Management
Tinea capitis (local treatment is usually unsuccessful)
- Local:
  - Apply Whitfield's® ointment or 1% clotrimazole cream (Canesten®) to the lesions.
  - It is not necessary to shave off the rest of the hair. Shampoo regularly with Betadine® or selenium sulphide.
  - Oral antibiotic if there is lymphadenopathy.
- In severe cases, give oral griseofulvin 10–15 mg/kg/24 hours for four to six weeks (contraindications are liver disease or sensitivity to the drug).

Tinea corporis / Tinea vesicolor
* Local:
  o Whitfield's® ointment (inexpensive); rub in four times daily until clear (may take several weeks).
or
  o 1% clotrimazole (Canesten®) or miconazole 2% (Daktarin®), ketoconazole (Nizcreme®) or econazole (Pevaryl®) may be used (all more expensive).
* Oral:
  o Griseofulvin by mouth for four weeks if lesions are extensive.

Note: It is important to tell parents that treatment takes a long time (six weeks plus), or they will go off and seek other forms of treatment.

Reasons for referral
Failure of one course of treatment. The diagnosis may need to be confirmed, using special techniques for demonstrating the fungus in the skin.

'Sandworm' (Cutaneous larva migrans, creeping eruption)
The larva of the dog hookworm, which enters the skin through cracks or abrasions, usually causes this. It is unable to complete its natural cycle in humans, and wanders aimlessly under the skin (1–2 cm per day). Most often seen around the anus, genitalia or feet. The typical lesions are S-shaped tracks under the skin.

Treatment
Local Thiabendazole (oral suspension) or tablets crushed with petroleum jelly can be used for extensive lesions. Self-limiting condition, as larva usually dies within weeks.

Seborrhoeic dermatitis
See Eczema, p. 292.

Scabies
Definition
A very itchy widespread skin rash caused by infestation with the mite *Sarcoptes scabiei*.

Cause

The female mite burrows into the skin where she lays eggs. These hatch into larvae in four to five days. They grow in the burrows and later emerge as adults who make new burrows. The cycle is repeated, and within a few weeks the infestation is extensive. After about one month of infestation, the mite body products and excreta induce an allergic reaction, which causes the rash.

Epidemiology

- Occurs at all ages from infancy. Mites are transmitted by direct contact between individuals involved and many household members are often simultaneously affected.
- More common where opportunities for regular bathing are poor and where living, and especially sleeping, conditions are overcrowded.

Clinical features

- Severe itching, especially at night and in warm conditions.
- Papular / vesicular rash, especially between fingers, on palms of hands, front of wrists, front fold of axilla, waistline, penis, and umbilicus. In infants, watery lesions are often seen, especially on face and feet.

Complications

- Secondary bacterial infection is very common, and presents as impetigo. If streptococcal, it may occasionally be complicated by acute glomerulonephritis.

Management

Children over three months and adults:
Use this regime for all household members:

- Cut fingernails.
- Wash well all over – this is most easily done in a hot bath.
- Dry well. Apply 1% gamma benzene hexachloride (cream or lotion) or benzyl benzoate lotion over the whole skin except face and head.
  Note: Get it into all skin folds, including the umbilicus.
- Let the lotion dry on the skin.
- Put the lotion on again as above.
- Put on clothes (need not change them).
- Do not wash for one day and night, and then wash all over. Put on clean clothes and use clean bed clothes and towels.
- May need to be repeated one week later.

Note: Give patients a simple instruction sheet. Warn them that this treatment will cause mild discomfort and a burning sensation where the benzyl benzoate is applied.
- Treat all affected family members at the same time.
- Linen and clothes must be washed in hot water.

Infants under three months:
Avoid gamma benzene hexachloride and benzyl benzoate as absorption may be dangerous in this age group.
Tetmosol® soap: Bath first and then use Tetmosol® soap to cover the whole body (not face) and allow to dry. Repeat next day. Then wash all clothes and bedding with the soap.
2,5% sulphur ointment: As an alternative, apply 2,5% sulphur ointment three times daily for three days.

For infected scabies:
- Treat as above, and then treat all infected areas with vioform in zinc ointment.
- If severe infection, oral antibiotics as per impetigo are needed.

Indications for referral:
Failure to respond to two courses of therapy.

Urticaria (Hives)
Definition
Sudden appearance of raised erythematous wheals, which may be localised or generalised, intensely itchy, or not itchy at all.

Causes
Due to a wide range of ingestants, contactants, injectants, inhalants, infections, physical factors, and systemic diseases.

Epidemiology
Up to 20% of people may experience urticaria at some stage.

Clinical features
Welts or wheals, which are well circumscribed with normal skin in-between the lesions. The rash tends to come and go and change its pattern over minutes. The wheals may appear singly or in crops.

Complications

May be associated with angioneurotic reactions in which the face, tongue, and sometimes the larynx swell up leading to dangerous airway obstruction.

Management

Symptomatic treatment with an antihistaminic such as promethazine (Phenergan®) or hydroxyzine (Aterax®).

Warts

Aetiology

All caused by the same viral agent; common in children.

Clinical features and management

Common warts

- Discrete, circular, papular lesions.
- Isolated or in crops; often on hands, but can be found anywhere.
- Often disappear spontaneously and so many home remedies are said to work.
- Treatment:
  - Local cauterisation by liquid nitrogen (painful) or a caustic pencil or podophyllin.

Plantar warts

- Same as above, but on soles of feet.
- Flat and painful due to pressure.
- Treatment:
  - 25% salicylic acid or podophyllin applied with extreme care to the wart only.

Flat warts

- Small, flat, and often extensive.
- Mainly hands and face; often follow scratch lines.
- Usually difficult to treat due to extent.

Chapter 17

Common surgical problems

Gastrointestinal conditions

Acute abdomen

This is a surgical emergency.

Features suggestive of an acute abdomen are:
- Sudden onset of continuous or colicky abdominal pain with or without vomiting which, in turn, may be bile-stained or not.
- Pain lasting more than one hour.
- Child waking at night with severe pain.

Causes
- Intestinal obstruction.
- Peritonitis.
- Strangulated hernia.

Management
- Refer to hospital urgently.
- Pass a nasogastric tube.
- Commence IV therapy.
- Keep nil per mouth.
- As urgent surgery may be necessary, parent to accompany to sign consent.

Early diagnosis and referral is of utmost importance. A delay of a few hours may significantly alter the prognosis.

The important danger signs are:
- Bile-stained vomiting.
- Distension of abdomen.
- Guarding on palpation.
- Tenderness on direct palpation, or 'rebound' tenderness (peritoneal irritation).
- Muscular rigidity.
- Abdominal mass.

- Blood in stool.
- Associated shock.

It is essential to examine the chest, urine, and measure the blood pressure in these cases. Basal pneumonia or pleurisy and pyelonephritis may present with abdominal pain, but without tenderness on palpation. Sometimes acute gastroenteritis presents with abdominal distension and vomiting, the diarrhoea starting a few hours later. In these cases the abdomen will not be tender, although the older child may complain of intermittent pain (cramps). Cramps in young children are uncommon.

Ileus (Paralytic)
Presents as abdominal distension with absent bowel sounds and minimal pain, except in the presence of peritonitis or ischaemic bowel.

Occurs as:
- Complication of acute infections:
  - Infants: Severe diarrhoea.
  - Older child: Perforated appendicitis (peritonitis).
  - Start of severe toxaemia / septicaemia.
- Electrolyte imbalance (hypokalaemia).
- Uraemia.
- Post-abdominal surgery / laparotomy.

Management
- Nasogastric tube for drainage.
- IV therapy – correct shock if present.
- Treat associated sepsis as necessary.
- Refer urgently.

Vomiting
Any vomiting in a baby, infant or child which is of sudden onset, persistent, copious, with or without bile, must be regarded as being due to a surgical condition until proven otherwise. Urgent referral is necessary, especially if vomitus is bile-stained.

Neonatal

It is important to recognise neonatal surgical emergencies as early as possible. These children usually present with signs (the so-called red flags) signaling danger:

- Excessive salivation.
- Abdominal distension.
- Bile-stained vomiting.
- Abdominal mass.
- Failure to pass meconium during the first 36 hours of life.
- Inability to void urine.

All such cases should be referred urgently.

Oesophageal atresia
See Newborn, p. 113.

Pyloric stenosis
Congenital hypertrophy of the pyloric muscle causing obstruction to gastric outflow.

Epidemiology
- Occurs more frequently in male infants.
- Age two to ten weeks (not present at birth).
- Rare in preterm infants.

Clinical features
- Classically, projectile vomiting; but this need not always be the pattern.
- Dehydration.
- Loss of weight and failure to thrive.
- Constipation.
- Metabolic alkalosis (if blood acid base status available) due to loss of acid from stomach with ongoing vomiting.

Diagnosis
- History and nature of vomiting can strongly suggest diagnosis.
- Inspection of the abdomen may show waves of peristalsis passing from left to right in the upper abdomen or in the epigastrium.
- On abdominal palpation, a firm 'tumour' (size of an acorn) can be felt in the epigastrium during a feed.
- Confirmed by ultrasound or barium meal.

Management
- IV fluid if dehydrated.
- Keep nil per mouth.
- Refer urgently for surgery.

Genito-urinary tract conditions

Balanitis

Inflammation of the glans penis and the prepuce, which occurs mostly when the prepuce is not or cannot be retracted to ensure proper cleanliness.

Treatment

- Prevention by frequent nappy changes and good genital hygiene.
- Mild cases respond to local cleaning and topical antibiotics.
- Severe cases may need systemic antibiotics.
- Circumcision may be indicated.

Circumcision

The prepuce is always adherent to the glans during the first year of life. Forcible retraction should be avoided until spontaneous separation occurs, usually in the second year but occasionally delayed for three to four years. There is therefore no need to retract the foreskin in the first few years of life. It is not an indication for circumcision. Under no circumstances must it be forcibly retracted, as this can result in paraphimosis.

Indications for circumcision

- Strong religious or tribal beliefs.
- Occurrence of phimosis or paraphimosis.
- Recurrent balanitis.
- Strong desire on part of parents, if cannot be dissuaded.
- The medical reason for circumcision is severe phimosis, which is caused by repeated episodes of balanitis.

Complications

- Local damage to glans – meatal stenosis.
- Severe haemorrhage (frenular artery).
- Complications associated with general anaesthesia.
- Infection and death from septicaemia arising from circumcision under unhygienic conditions.

Circumcision is never indicated because of a foreskin that is 'too long'.

Hernias

Inguinal hernia in boys
Seen as a swelling or 'rupture' in the inguinal area; can extend right into the scrotum.

Clinical features
- Occurs more frequently in infants who were born preterm.
- May be visible at all times; or may only become apparent with increased abdominal pressure when child cries, coughs, or on sitting or standing up.
- Usually causes no pain.

The diagnosis can often be made on history alone.

Management
Must be referred as soon as diagnosed, due to the ever-present risk of strangulation of bowel or gonad. Surgery is the only form of management, and is done as soon as possible after diagnosis.

Inguinal hernia in girls
- Occurs less commonly than in boys.
- The clinical picture is the same as in boys.
- Ovary may herniate into the sac.
- Urgent referral necessary due to danger of strangulation; possibility of associated intersex if hernias are bilateral.

Fluid hernia
During the first 12 months or so, most fluid hernias (often incorrectly called hydrocoeles) cure themselves. If they are very large or persist beyond this age, they must be referred, as they progress to become inguinal hernias and rarely disappear spontaneously thereafter. A fluid hernia can be transilluminated as the fluid 'lights up'.

Umbilical hernia
True umbilical hernia is very common, and usually resolves spontaneously within the first year of life, but closure may continue into the second and third years. There is no need for strapping or the use of a truss. Surgery is usually not considered before the age of two to five years.

Genital

Hypospadias

Clinical features

- The urethral meatus opens proximal to its usual position:
  - Along the shaft of the penis.
  - Between the scrotal folds.
  - On the perineum.
- The prepuce is deficient on the underside of the penis.
- Chordae (the penis is curved downwards).
- Inability to direct the urinary stream.

Management

- All such cases must be referred for assessment.
- Surgical correction is usually done at three to four years of age, if the flow of urine is not in a forward direction.
- Full assessment is important, as apparent hypospadias may occur in a virilised female and early diagnosis is essential. If both testes are not in the scrotum, intersex must be suspected and the infant referred for assessment immediately.

Note: No child with a hypospadias should be circumcised, as the prepuce skin may be required for surgical correction.

Paraphimosis

The prepuce is in a retracted position, with constriction and fibrosis around the shaft of the penis. This may occur suddenly on retracting a fibrosed prepuce and may be manually reducible or irreducible requiring surgery. Surgical treatment takes the form of circumcision.

Phimosis

This is stenosis of the opening of the prepuce with constriction of the foreskin, which makes retraction impossible. Often follows excoriation and infection from poor nappy care. May require incision or circumcision. If mild, may respond to 1% hydrocortisone cream locally for one week.

Torsion of testis

Any acute painful swelling in the scrotum should be referred immediately, before testis is lost due to ischaemia.

Undescended testes

Common condition. Found in 4% of newborns. As testes may take about three months before they reach their permanent descended position, diagnosis of undescended testis only made after this age.

Cause of an 'empty scrotum':
- Retractile testes:
  - Protective withdrawal phenomenon (cremasteric reflex).
  - Need to be 'stroked' down into the scrotum.
- Undescended testes:
  - Abdominal (retroperitoneal).
  - In inguinal canal – partially descended.
  - In a high scrotal position.
- Ectopic testes:
  - In an abnormal position outside the line of descent.
- Agenesis of the testes.
- Atrophy of testes.

Management
- Make a correct diagnosis:
  - Warm hands when examining (retractile).
  - Stroke down inguinal canal with thumb.
  - Get patient to 'squat' while examining.
  - Examine after a warm bath.
- Refer after one year of age for surgical correction.

Complications
- Malignancy (increased incidence later in life).
- Sterility, especially if bilateral (later in life).
- Torsion.
- Associated hernia.
- Psychological effect.
- Trauma to testes.

Musculoskeletal disorders

Abnormal gait

In children, this can arise from:
- Painful conditions:
  - Trauma / fracture.

- o Soft tissue inflammation.
- o Osteomyelitis.
- o Tumours.
- o Avascular necrosis of epiphysis.
- o Spinal causes.
- Diseases of the CNS:
  - o Cerebral palsy.
  - o Ataxia.
- Diseases of muscle:
  - o Muscular dystrophy.
- Joint disorders:
  - o Congenital dislocation of hip.
  - o Ankylosis.
  - o Joint instability.
  - o Contractures.
  - o Perthes' Disease (hip).
  - o Irritable hip.
- Bone deformity:
  - o Leg length discrepancy.
  - o Coxa vara (bow legs).
  - o Congenital bone abnormalities.
- Functional states:
  - o Hysteria.
- Mimicry:
  - o Many conditions presenting with abnormal gait are non-surgical, and careful assessment is required.

Bow legs / toeing in / knock knees
Bow legs

The legs of the normal older infant and toddler often appear bowed, causing parental anxiety. This is almost always a self-rectifying condition, requiring no treatment. If there is severe bowing, the child must be referred for the exclusion of bone disease or severe rickets. Sometimes a child, who at nine to 12 months has mild bow legs, may develop knock knees when he or she is two to three years old. The majority of children will grow out of a knock-knee deformity by the age of six years, as part of normal development and as the muscles strengthen.

Bow legs usually require no treatment, but if there is evidence of abnormal weight-bearing as shown by abnormal shoe wear, the child should be referred for assessment.

Toeing in

Most cases of toeing in (or out) will correct themselves spontaneously. However, if severe or if causing clumsy gait, the child should be referred, as the condition may be due to torsion of the long bones which may require corrective surgery.

Knock knees

Knock knees commencing in older children (seven to eight years), or persisting beyond this time, are often a non-resolving condition and may require corrective surgery. Such cases should, therefore, be referred.

Club foot *(See Newborn, p. 112)*

Congenital 'club foot' usually occurs as an isolated abnormality, but must be distinguished from a similar deformity secondary to other conditions such as meningomyelocele, cerebral palsy, etc. There is often a family history of club foot. The severity of the condition varies from mild to one of severe deformity. Best results are obtained when treatment is started shortly after birth. The normal baby has pliable feet and any mild deformity can be overcome by gently twisting the foot into a normal position. If there is stiffness and passive correction is not obtained, then club foot is diagnosed and the child should be referred for treatment. This usually consists of manipulation and splintage with serial plaster of Paris casts. If correction is not obtained over a period of three to six months, surgical release may be necessary.

Congenital dislocation of hip (CDH) *(See Newborn, p. 111)*

This is a common condition with a familial tendency. Early diagnosis is extremely important, as simple treatment at this stage usually leads to a child with normal hips.

Until the baby is seen for assessment, thick double nappies can be used, as these tend to encourage a 'frog' position.

Flat foot

The diagnosis of flat foot as a cause of symptoms in a child is almost always wrong. Treatment of flat feet is hardly ever necessary. The pad of fat under the feet of the young child gives the impression of a flat foot. The only untroubled person is the child, but the apparent condition causes considerable anxiety in parents, teachers, and doctors.

Only a small percentage of children with postural flat feet will continue to have flat feet. If the inner side of the shoe or heel is showing wear, the child should be referred for assessment.

Children with flat feet should be referred if the following occur:

- **Spasmodic flat foot:** Inversion of the foot is prominent, and causes pain with spasm in the tendons on the lateral side of the ankle. Usually this signifies a congenital bony deformity in the foot that may require surgery. The condition usually becomes painful only in older children.
- **Severe flat foot:** If associated with poor gait or especially weakness of the legs, the foot deformity may be caused by other conditions such as neuro-muscular disorders.
- **Rocker-bottom foot:** Here the longitudinal arch of the foot is reversed. In the infant, it may be due to birth trauma or to neuro-muscular disorders, or occasionally it may be due to a congenital vertical talus. This condition is also found in certain syndromes, for example trisomy 18.

Limp

Definition

Any abnormality of gait. It is commonly seen and frequently painless. There are innumerable causes, and children should be referred if there is no local evidence of, or history of trauma. Possible causes range from central nervous system, spinal, hip, leg or foot pathology. (See also Abnormal gait, p. 311).

Osteomyelitis

Definition

Bacterial infection of bone.

Causative organism

- Commonly *Staphylococcus aureus*.
- Also streptococci and certain Gram-negative organisms.
- Tuberculosis.

Epidemiology

- Occurs at any age, but is more common between three to 12 years.
- Twice as likely to occur in boys as in girls.

Clinical features

- Early symptoms vary from 12 to 24 hours.
- Child may present with a limp or not using a hand / arm.
- Painful limb with tenderness over the metaphysis of a bone.
- Fever and systemic signs of toxicity.

- Subacute illness with local pain at the involved site.
- X-ray changes only occur after 10–14 days, so early X-rays look normal, but serve as a control.

Management
- Refer to confirm diagnosis.
- Drainage.
- Antibiotics – cloxacillin (for sensitive organism).
- Immobilisation.

Differential diagnosis of an 'acute painful limb'
- Osteomyelitis.
- Septic arthritis.
- Cellulitis / local abscess.
- Acute rheumatic fever.
- Scurvy.
- Incomplete fracture / trauma / soft tissue bruising.
- Malignancies, for example leukaemia, bone tumours, or secondary deposits.

Scoliosis
Definition
Lateral curvature of the spine. Due to abnormality of the spine, which is either structural or postural. It is more frequently found in adolescent girls.

Clinical features
Back towards examiner:
The normal spine is straight when viewed from behind. With scoliosis present:
- Head and neck base are off centre.
- Uneven shoulder elevation.
- Obvious spinal curvature.
- Uneven shoulder blades.
- Uneven waist creases.

Facing examiner:
- Uneven hip prominence.
- Unequal arm to body space.

Forward bend:
- Ribs more prominent on one side.

Exclude underlying chest or lung pathology

Treatment
- Early detection; refer all cases.
- Conservative with spinal brace after assessment. Physiotherapy alone is usually ineffective.
- Operative with spine fixation – various methods.

Torticollis ('Crick neck')
Mild torticollis may be due to intrauterine positioning and can be cured by stretching exercises. Other common causes for torticollis are fibrosis of the sternomastoid muscle, cervical hemivertebra, or imbalance of the ocular muscles. It is important to recognise the type, as each requires specific treatment. If the neck is normal and the sternomastoid muscle of normal texture, ocular imbalance is then the most likely cause. Refer for full assessment.

Neurological disorders

Hydrocephalus
The majority of infants with large heads suffer from an imbalance between the production and absorption of CSF. The head circumference should always be measured when a baby is examined. Determine the cause if it is markedly larger than expected for the weight and length percentiles. Not all infants with enlargement of the head require surgery. Referral is mandatory if there is deviation from the normal growth curves. If fontanelle is open, ultrasound is an accurate, non-invasive investigation.

Meningomyelocele / spina bifida (See also p. 113)
Any child with abnormalities of the skin overlying the vertebral column (meningomyelocele, patch of dark hair, pigmented naevus, haemangioma, lipoma, dimple), or one with obvious skeletal spinal abnormalities (spina bifida) should be referred for neurosurgical opinion. The important associated problems are hydrocephalus, urinary retention, and paralysed lower limbs. Risk of recurrence can be reduced with folic acid supplements before and during early pregnancy.

Trauma / infection

Abscess

Definition

Staphylococcal infection of the skin with the formation of a tense, painful swelling containing pus.

Cause

The staphylococci enter the deeper layers of the skin, either through a previously damaged area, or through a hair follicle.

Epidemiology

- Diabetics are especially prone to developing abscesses, so check urine for glucose in anyone who has repeated boils.
- Poor hygiene.
- Members of some households tend to be carriers of the responsible staphylococcus. This may be the reason why several members of a household develop abscesses simultaneously.

Clinical features

- A painful area of swelling and redness, which gradually develops a central point of softness. Boils of the perineal area tend to occur in crops.
- There may be malaise and fever.
- The local draining lymph glands are often swollen.
- The boil may later discharge spontaneously and eventually heal.
- Extremely painful, especially if in nose or ear.

Management

In general, the management of local infections is based on:

- Rest or immobilisation of the affected area.
- Appropriate antibiotics as required.
- Drainage of pus and excision of dead tissue.

Before the abscess becomes fluctuant:

- Antibiotics are seldom needed, except in malnourished children.
- Treat pain with an analgesic (e.g. paracetamol).

When fluctuation occurs, this is indicative of pus formation and the abscess needs to be drained. If this cannot be done locally, refer for incision and drainage. Local anaesthesia does not work effectively in the presence of pus. Once the abscess has been drained, systemic cloxacillin may hasten the healing process.

Burns

Burns are the result of skin trauma due to hot liquids, fire, electricity or chemicals.

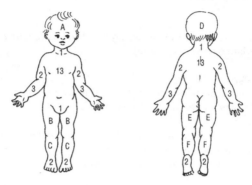

Figure 17.1 Burns assessment and tabulation figures (Body surface area percentages)

Region	Age (years)				
	0	1	5	10	15
A/D head	10	9	7	6	5
B/E thigh	3	3	4	5	5
C/F leg	2	3	3	3	3

Body surface area (percentage) according to age

Major burns

The following are regarded as major burns, and these cases should all be admitted to hospital:

- More than 5% of skin surface burned in children under two years.
- More than 10% of skin surface burned in children over two years.
- Burns of face, hands, feet, perineum or flexures, and circumferential burns.
- All infected burns.
- Burns not healed within 14 days.

- All electric current burns.
- All deep burns. A deep burn has the following characteristics:
  ○ There is no pain on pinprick over the central area of the burn.
  ○ The burn feels hard and leathery.
  ○ It has a white or black appearance and has no blister formation.
  ○ Does not blanch on pressure, that is, there is no circulation.

Minor burns
Burns over a small area without any of the above-mentioned features.

Treatment
Major burns
- Cool the burned area immediately with cold water after removing the heat source. It may be possible to do this by holding the affected part under cold water for ten minutes.
- Cover with a clean bandage or cloth.
- Do not apply anything to the burned surface.
- Commence IV fluids if the burn covers more than 15% of the body surface, and the journey may take longer than two hours. (Ringer's lactate or Plasmalyte B®: volume 20 ml per kg body weight over one to two hours).
- Pass a nasogastric tube and empty the stomach to prevent vomiting.
- Transfer to hospital as soon as above is done. Give analgesics if any delay in transfer.

Minor burns
- Immediately cool the burned area with cold water (as above).
- Clean the burn with water. Wash, do not scrub.
- Cover with Povidone Iodine cream, dry gauze, and bandage. Change the dressing twice daily, or use Flamazine® cream if available and dress every second day.
- Burns should heal within 14 days.
- Panado® for pain.
- Do not use prophylactic antibiotics.

Dog bites
These are treated in the same way as any other penetrating injury. Clean the wound and prescribe an antibiotic if the wound is dirty or had to be sutured. A booster dose of tetanus toxoid is desirable, unless this has been given within the previous three years. A dog bite on the face or hands is better dealt with by someone with surgical experience.

Fractures / severe sprains
Caused by
- Violence, direct or indirect.
- Disease – pathological fractures are not uncommon in children (e.g. osteogenesis imperfecta).

Fractures can be:
- Simple, that is, closed.
- Compound – bone is in contact with the air. This is either due to bone piercing outwards through skin, or an external object piercing inwards.

Clinical diagnosis
If there is pain in a limb, even small children will point to the site of pain. The suspicion of a fracture may be confirmed by local tenderness and pain on gentle passive pressure and movement of the area. If a fracture is suspected, X-rays should be taken. The fracture may be displaced and will then require reduction and immobilisation.

At day centres / clinics:
Greenstick or non-displaced simple fractures can be treated, but only if there is no clinical deformity or temperature. Movement, sensation, and colour of the limb must be normal and the pulse must always be palpable beyond the level of the fracture.

Fractures of the humerus, radius, ulna, tibia, and fibula can be managed without referral if the above criteria have been met. Femoral fractures are best treated in traction and should be referred.

Treatment
Note: A child should be reassessed immediately if, after immobilisation, he or she complains of the sensation of pins and needles, constant and progressive pain, or circulatory changes in the immobilised limb. This may indicate vascular compromise. If in doubt, remove or split the plaster of Paris (POP).

Humerus
Light POP U-Slab over plasterwool and crêpe bandage. Support with a collar and cuff and the limb under clothing. Check colour of limb, pulse, and temperature daily for three days.

Forearm

Light POP slab over plasterwool and firm crêpe bandage. Support with collar and cuff. Check daily as above.

Note: Check wrist movement. If there is any limitation, suspect a slipped radial epiphysis and refer to hospital.

Tibia and fibula

POP backslab over plasterwool and firm crêpe bandage. Not to bear weight on leg for three weeks. The child will start walking on his or her own accord when the fracture is united and pain-free. Warn parents that they must return immediately if:

- Any severe swelling develops.
- The child complains of severe burning sensation.
- A small baby becomes irritable.
- A change of colour or temperature in extremities occurs.

Always give analgesics for about three days, for example paracetamol (Panado®).

Always refer the following to hospital

A child with:

- Any injury involving a joint or very near to a joint.
- Any injury causing deformity, loss of warmth in limb, change in colour, severe swelling, loss of sensation, loss of pulse beyond injury or loss of movement.
- Any severe swelling with redness (inflammation), increased local temperature of limb, local blistering, and intense pain accompanied by pyrexia, general toxicity, and inability to bear weight or a high ESR. These signs could mean an underlying osteitis.
- Any head or neck injuries (stabilise the head and neck before transfer).
- Hand or foot injuries and fractures often involve small bones of the wrist or feet and are not obvious. Unless fractures involving joints are treated correctly from the beginning, post-traumatic arthritis may occur later.

Problems

Repeated fractures:

- Consider osteogenesis imperfecta or other pathological fractures, for example related to malignant bone tumour or due to other tumour secondaries.

- Non-accidental injury / child abuse.
- Osteoporosis, for example a deficiency disease such as rickets.

The history is important:
- Suspect a pathological fracture if the child was running, kneeling or walking, felt a sudden pain, and then fell.
- Severity of injury out of proportion to fracture.
- If child is known to have malignant disease.
- Suspect child abuse if there are two or more fractures, other signs of assault, and the history does not fit the findings.

In a limping child complaining of pain in the knee, always check the hip, as pain is often referred from hip to knee.

Splinting: If children have to be transferred in a hurry, the body can act as a very good splint, for example forearms together, legs together or arm to chest wall. Remember to pad any prominences, for example knees, wrists, elbows before securing together.

Lacerations / fingertip injuries / amputations
Principles of management of any laceration
- Local anaesthesia.
- Wound irrigation.
- Debridement.
- Proper closure (sterile technique).
- If a clean wound needs suturing, this should be done within six hours of the injury.
- If there has been delay in presentation and suturing is necessary, give antibiotic cover in addition. Wounds must be cleaned of all foreign material.
- Any wound which enters another plane, that is, into a muscle or deeper structures, must be referred.
- Large gaping septic wounds must always be referred. They will require antibiotics and suturing after appropriate debridement (cleaning up).
- Any penetrating wound made by a sharp thin object must be referred if it involves the head, chest, abdomen or is over a joint. In these cases, the extent of internal damage may not be clinically apparent. Do not probe the wound.
- Dirty and penetrating wounds must be carefully cleaned and an injection of tetanus toxoid given. It can be given even after a week's delay.

Fingertip injury
Commonly seen and results in loss of a part due to crushing or slicing injury, or in partial amputation of tip. Do not remove nail or tissue before referring.

In young children:
Debridement and trimming of skin and bone is often all that is needed. No graft is required unless the line of section is very oblique.

In older children:
Refer for primary closure or a free graft or local flap, which may be required to accomplish anatomical and functional reconstruction.

Management of amputated part of limb:
Pack in ice and send patient to hospital.

Hand injuries
Any significant hand injury should be referred to hospital for optimal management to ensure full anatomical and functional recovery.

Head trauma / concussion (See Central nervous system, p. 130)
Refer the child to hospital immediately if after a head injury there is evidence of amnesia, vomiting, convulsions, confusion, depressed level of consciousness, or the presence of blood or CSF from ear or nose.

If there was any loss of consciousness or a seizure, no matter how brief, the child should also be referred for assessment. In other cases not referred, the parents must be warned to be alert for the onset of increasing drowsiness, headache, vomiting, undue irritability, incessant crying, or loss of interest in toys and play. If any of these develop, the child should be referred immediately, as there may be intracranial bleeding. Associated skull fractures, especially if depressed, should be referred immediately.

Life-saving measures may have to be carried out at the time of injury or soon afterwards. The patient must be moved carefully as his or her neck may be broken. (See the ABCD of resuscitation below and pp. 338–340.)

A Airway	– patent
B Breathing	– adequate or needs support (Ambubag)
C Cardiac / circulation	– stop external bleeding
	– cardiac resuscitation
	– treatment of shock
D Diagnosis	

Timing of surgical procedures

The optimum time to correct an abnormality is determined by the condition.

Immediate / urgent group

Trauma, acute infections, abdominal emergencies, acute scrotal conditions, neonatal emergencies.

Intermediate group (No undue delay)

Inguinal hernias, CNS abnormalities, skeletal abnormalities (club foot, CDH).

Elective group (optimum age)

Condition	Optimal age for surgery
Cleft lip and palate	3–4 months
Cleft palate	Variable 12–15 months or 5–10 days
Circumcision	Post nappy-wearing age
Hypospadias	2–4 years
Skeletal abnormalities	Depending on abnormality
Strabismus (congenital)	Refer for occlusion treatment; surgery 12–15 months
Strabismus (acquired)	When diagnosed, refer for full assessment
Umbilical hernia	2 years
Undescended testes	2 years

Miscellaneous

Bed rest
There are few conditions in paediatrics which require absolute bed rest. This is often used by the medical profession as the great placebo. Unnecessary confinement to bed must be avoided, unless the child wants to be in bed or needs to be in bed for specific medical reasons, for example rheumatic fever.

Child abuse and neglect
Other terms used are battered baby syndrome and non-accidental injury.

Types of abuse
These may be physical, sexual, emotional, nutritional, and wilful neglect.

Suspect abuse if:
- The child has an unexplained injury.
- The child states that injury has been inflicted.
- There is evidence of previous injury or neglect.
- The parent / caretaker gives a history inappropriate to the injury.
- The child has associated marked behavioural disorders.
- The parent / caretaker has delayed unduly before seeking advice.
- The parent / caretaker manifests emotional or social maladjustment.
- The parent presents for help with 'trivial' problem. This is often a sign of 'plea for help' by parents.

Investigations
- Full history: Note home and family interrelationships.
- Full physical examination.
- Radiological skeletal survey.
- FBC and clotting profile to exclude bleeding disorders.
- In sexual abuse, vaginal swabs, VDRL, and HIV testing.
- Pregnancy test in menarchial girls to exclude existing pregnancy.

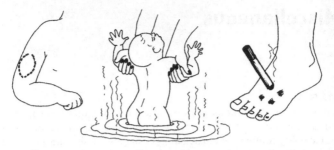

bite   hot water   cigarette

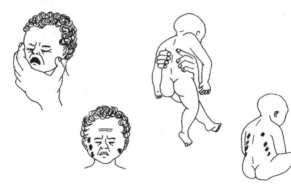

fingertip bruises

Figure 18.1 Forms of non-accidental injury

Differential diagnosis
- Bruising due to blood disease.
- 'Mongolian' pigmentation (blue naevus) on the lower back of young infants can resemble bruises.
- Periosteal elevation in scurvy and syphilis.

Management
- Active intervention to prevent re-injury.
- May need hospitalisation and medical treatment.
- Refer to child protection services of the police or child welfare agency.

- Accurate documentation of clinical signs or injuries with sketches and photographs.
- In South Africa it is a criminal offence to not report child abuse.
- In sexual abuse, the child will need antiretroviral prophylaxis if seen within 72 hours.
- Pregnancy prophylaxis in menarchial girls.
- Management is best done by a multidisciplinary team with experience in child abuse.

Role of the nurse
If a medical doctor is not available or referral is not possible, a professional nurse who has been trained appropriately can manage all types of child abuse and can testify in court.

Prevention of Family Violence Act no 133 of 1993 (section 4) South Africa
In this act it is stated that 'any person who examines, treats, attends to, advises, instructs or cares for any child in circumstances which ought to give rise to the reasonable suspicion that such child has been ill-treated, or suffers from any injury the probable cause of which was deliberate, shall immediately report such circumstances: a) To a police official; or b) to a commissioner of child welfare or a social worker...'

Child Care Amendment Act 96 of 1996
The Act states in section no 15 (Amendment of section 42 of Child Care Act 74 of 1983) that 'Notwithstanding the provisions of any other law every dentist, medical practitioner, nurse, social worker or teacher, or any person employed by or managing a children's home, place of care or shelter, who examines, attends or deals with any child in circumstances giving rise to the suspicion that that child has been ill-treated, or suffers from any injury, single or multiple, the cause of which probably might have been deliberate, or suffers from a nutritional deficiency disease, shall immediately notify the Director-General (now Director of Welfare) or any officer designated by him or her for the purpose of this section, of those circumstances.'

Hypothyroidism (Cretinism)
Syndrome appearing in infancy as a result of deficiency of thyroid hormone during fetal or early life. Clinical features are usually not present at birth. If not detected early, hypothyroidism causes severe irreversible mental retardation. This is an avoidable tragedy.

Clinical features
- Prolonged neonatal jaundice.
- Constipation.
- Apathetic and feeds poorly.
- Cool skin with hypothermia.
- Thick, mottled, and dry skin.
- Enlarged protruding tongue.
- Broad face with coarse features and puffiness.

Management
- Early detection. May be screened for by measuring TSH routinely in cord blood at birth. The incidence of congenital hypothyroidism is 1:5 000 to 1:20 000 in different communities.
- Refer for laboratory investigation of TSH, T4, and thyroid scan to confirm clinical diagnosis.
- Daily replacement thyroxine treatment for life is best given through endocrine clinics.

Diabetes mellitus
Diabetes mellitus is a chronic but controllable metabolic disease affecting the utilisation of carbohydrate, protein, and fat.

It is characterised by
- Insufficient insulin production.
- An abnormally high blood glucose level (hyperglycaemia).
- Glycosuria (with or without ketonuria).

Types of diabetes
- Juvenile onset diabetes (JOD) which is insulin-dependent and often hereditary.
- Secondary to other conditions, for example destruction of the pancreas in cystic fibrosis.
- Maturity onset diabetes (MOD). Usually in adults. May respond to oral drugs which stimulate the pancreas. Associated with a family history and obesity.

Clinical features
- Polydypsia (increased thirst).
- Polyuria (glucose diuresis).
- Fatigue, muscle weakness, and loss of weight because of increased fat and protein breakdown.

- Increased appetite.
- Blurring of vision as a result of disturbed fluid balance caused by polyuria.
- Skin becomes dry and itching with pruritus vulvae. Fungal infections and boils are common.
- May present in coma.

Management
- Early detection by screening the population at risk.
- Think of the diagnosis in children with polyuria, polydipsia or weight loss.
- Refer urgently for medical management and control.
- Regular attendance at hospital or diabetic clinic.
- Use of the diabetic information, guidance, and counselling services.
- Attendance of holiday camps for diabetic children organised by Diabetic Associations.
- Education of child and parents.
- Insulin by injection or oral antidiabetic drugs (adults mainly).

Complications
These are greatly reduced if adequate control is achieved.
- Diabetic coma: Refer urgently: start normal saline infusion.
- Hypoglycaemic coma: This is extremely dangerous; give IV glucose and refer urgently.
- Lowered resistance giving rise to sepsis.
- The eyes may be affected, for example diabetic cataracts, glaucoma, and retinal changes may lead to blindness.
- Diabetic gangrene which may be started by trauma and aggravated by cold and infection.
- Diabetic dwarfism in JOD children who have been poorly controlled. The child is short, fat, and physically immature.

Down syndrome (Trisomy 21 syndrome)
Definition
Due to the presence of extra material from the no. 21 chromosome. Usually due to chromosomal non-disjunction in the ovum, which is more common in older women. This results in three, instead of two, no. 21 chromosomes (trisomy 21). The other rarer causes are translocation and mosaicism.

- Mental retardation
- Hypotonia
- Craniofacial abnormalities
  ○ Flat occiput
  ○ Almond eyes
  ○ Epicanthic folds
  ○ Brushflield spots
- Cardiac defects
- Duodenal atresia
- Hand abnormalities
  ○ Single palmar crease
  ○ Short, incurved little finger
  ○ Abnormal dermaglyphics
- Foot abnormalities
  ○ Sandal gap

Figure 18.2 Down syndrome: Clinical features

Clinical features

- Typical facial appearance with epicanthic folds, slanting eyes, flat nasal bridge, protruding tongue, and small ears.
- Round head with flat occiput.
- Muscular hypotonia.
- Feeding difficulties.
- Short and broad hands and feet with single palmar creases, short incurving fifth fingers, and a gap between first and second toes (sandal gap).
- Retarded physical and mental development. Become placid children.
- Associated congenital abnormalities, for example cardiac septal defects and duodenal atresia.
- Incidence of infection and leukaemia is higher than for the general population.

Prevention

Ideally all pregnant women of 35 years or more should have an early ultrasound scan and amniocentesis during the first trimester in order to offer medical termination if necessary.

Management

- Avoid pregnancy over 34 years.
- Genetic counselling.

- Education and stimulation to achieve maximum ability.
- Contact local Down Syndrome Association if available.
- Symptomatic and supportive.
- Use of amniocentesis in further pregnancies.

Fever
Definition
Axillary temperature above 37 °C or an oral temperature above 37,5 °C. Use a digital rather than mercury thermometer. Fever is usually a sign of infection or inflammation and is not a diagnosis in itself. Always look for the underlying cause.

A high fever in a child under six years may cause a convulsion.

Management in all cases regardless of cause
- Remove excessive clothing or blankets.
- Paracetamol (Panado®).
- Give extra water to drink.
- Cool the child with fanning and tepid sponging. Advise mother of these measures.
- Look for the cause, especially pneumonia, otitis media, tonsillitis or urinary tract infection. The child may also be incubating a viral infectious disease. Treat the cause.
- If no cause obvious, lumbar puncture may be indicated in young infant. Refer.

Fetal alcohol syndrome (FAS)
- Alcohol ingestion by pregnant mothers is an increasing and serious problem. There is a need to educate people about the effects of alcohol during pregnancy on the unborn baby.
- Fetal alcohol syndrome is one of the most common avoidable causes of intellectual disability.

Aetiology
Alcohol acts as a teratogen, that is, an environmental 'toxic' agent that causes abnormal development. With raised levels of blood alcohol intake during pregnancy, there is a risk of abnormal embryonic and fetal development.

Clinical features
These may include:
- Low birth weight due to preterm delivery and fetal growth restriction.

- Microcephaly and underweight for gestational age.
- Mental and physical retardation postnatally.
- Typical facial features with short palpebral fissures, epicanthic folds, broad depressed nasal bridge, and flattened (thin) upper lip.
- Cardiac and limb defects common.

Treatment
- Prevention: 'When you drink, your unborn child does too'.
- Education regarding the effects of alcohol.
- Identify 'drinkers' among pregnant women.
- Support and encouragement is needed to modify excessive alcohol intake in pregnant mothers.

Growing pains
This term is inaccurate, as limb pains often occur at periods when there is no rapid growth. They are more frequent after exertion and fatigue. They are mainly confined to the lower limbs, to the calf and thigh muscles. They are not joint pains, and are not associated with underlying organic disease such as rheumatic fever. Reassurance is the main form of management, as the cause is benign. The condition is very real but poorly understood.

Gynaecomastia
Fat boys often appear to have breast enlargement. This is due to fat and not breast tissue. Enlargement and tenderness of breast tissue in an adolescent boy is normal and does not require treatment apart from reassurance. Normal newborn infants often have enlarged breasts for a few weeks. In all other cases of breast enlargement, the testes should be examined and cases must be referred if testes are not of normal size.

Juvenile chronic arthritis (JCA)
Clinical features
- Persistent arthritis or systemic illness for more than six weeks.
- Many different patterns of presentation.
- Not uncommon.
- Occurs in children under the age of 16 years. Only 5% of chronic arthritis starts in childhood.

Cause
Unknown. Falls under 'hypersensitivity' or 'auto-immune' group of diseases.

Mode of onset

Systemic disease

- About 10% of cases.
- Fever.
- Rash.
- Lymphadenopathy, splenomegaly, and hepatomegaly.
- Pericarditis, pleuritis or peritonitis.

Polyarticular disease

- About 30% of cases.
- More than four joints involved, including small joints of hands.

Monoarticular or pauciarticular disease

- About 60% of cases.
- One of four large joints involved. Knee most commonly affected.
- About 20% of this group develop uveitis.

Diagnosis and management

- Clinical recognition and awareness.
- Exclude conditions which mimic it. Be careful of missing a septic arthritis.
- Refer all cases for definitive diagnosis.
- Laboratory investigation for collagen disorders.
- Synovial biopsy (sometimes indicated).

Treatment

- Indomethicin.
- Steroids and methotrexate therapy at a special clinic for managing JCA.

Prognosis

- Variable. Usually good in childhood. Team approach with doctor, physiotherapist, social worker, orthopaedic appliance technician, etc.
- Surgery may be required.

Sudden infant death syndrome (SIDS)

Definition

The sudden and unexpected death of an infant for a reason that remains unclear even after an autopsy.

Age and sex
- 80% of cases occur between one and six months.
- Peak age is two to four months.
- 60% boys and 40% girls.

Risk factors
- Preterm infants with history of apnoea.
- Underweight for gestational age infants.
- Cold weather.
- Lower socio-economic group.
- Maternal history of smoking.
- History of a sibling with SIDS.
- Sleeping prone.

Cause
While there is much confusion about the cause, it is suggested that some of the following are relevant:
- Prolonged respiratory pauses leading to apneoic spells.
- Abnormal upper airway function.
- Cardiac abnormalities.

Management of SIDS family
- Support and reassurance. Many parents feel guilty.
- Explanation.
- Follow-up.

Treatment of infants with near-miss or aborted SIDS
- Home monitoring with apnoea monitor if possible.
- Teach parents basic resuscitation with a mask and bag.
- Careful observation and awareness of risk factor. Need full investigation and assessment to exclude possible CNS, cardiac or metabolic factors.

Vulvovaginitis
A clear mucoid discharge from the vagina in the newborn baby or at the time of puberty is usually normal and no treatment is required. Mild vulvovaginitis will respond to simple hygiene, washing the affected part daily, and application of a barrier cream. Some cases respond to oestrogen cream. Purulent or offensive discharge requires a systemic antibiotic. A swab should be taken for culture before commencing antibiotic treatment. Non-bacterial causes include monilia and Trichomonas,

which will respond to mycostatin and metronidazole respectively. If discharge persists in spite of treatment, suspect a foreign body and refer. If the swab result reveals gonococcus or Gardnerella, the child must be referred to a centre for full assessment to exclude possible sexual abuse. This is an extremely delicate matter and must be handled with great care. Unsubstantiated accusations must not be made.

Chapter 19

Emergencies

Anaphylaxis

Definition

An acute, severe allergic reaction to drugs (especially penicillin), bee stings, foods (especially nuts), etc.

Clinical features

- Within a minute or less of exposure, the patient suddenly collapses with sweating, pallor, cold extremities, weak and rapid pulse, low or unrecordable blood pressure and drowsiness.
- There may be difficulty with breathing, wheezing, stridor, cyanosis or apnoea.
- Oedema, particularly of mouth and throat, or urticaria may occur.
- The child may die if not correctly and immediately managed.

Management

- Lie the patient flat.
- Give oxygen by face mask.
- Intramuscular adrenaline 0,01 ml/kg/dose (maximum 0,5 ml).
- Followed by Phenergan® IV (IM if unable to give IV) 0,5 mg/kg.
- Intravenous fluids if possible, such as Plasmalyte B® or normal saline, 20 ml/kg given fast. Continue until blood pressure returns to normal.
- Hydrocortisone 100 mg IV.
- Once condition has improved, refer to hospital urgently.

Cardiorespiratory resuscitation

The person who finds collapsed child must:

- Grab the resuscitation box if in hospital or clinic.
- Call for help.
- Start resuscitation immediately, using the 'ABCD' drill.

ABCD of resuscitation
A. Airway

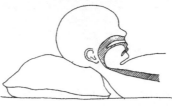

incorrect

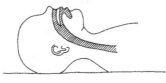

correct

Figure 19.1 Correct and incorrect position for airway

- Position patient with head back and hold jaw forward.
- Clear tongue and vomitus with fingers.
- Suction when available.

B. Breathing
- If not breathing well, give bag and mask ventilation using rapid and shallow inflations. Use large green inflating bag with medium mask for

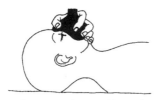

a) correct application of facemask

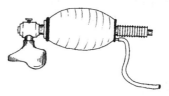

(b) ventilation bag and mask

Figure 19.2 (a) Artificial ventilation (b) Ventilation bag and mask

all patients. Small bag is intended for small children with endotracheal tubes or tracheostomies.

- If the chest does not move well, insert oral airway.
- Add oxygen as soon as available.
- All unconscious patients to be nursed on their side when breathing on their own.
- Mouth-to-mouth (or nose) resuscitation is potentially dangerous as this may carry the risk of transmitting HIV, especially if blood is present.

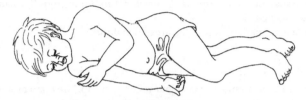

Figure 19.3 Positioning of unconscious patient

C. Cardiac

- If no pulse is felt (carotid, femoral or brachial) as soon as the lungs are ventilated, cardiac massage is required.
- In infants, use both hands to encircle the chest, thumbs compress the sternum towards backbone about 100/minute.
- In older children, use both hands together to press middle and lower sternum towards backbone, with child lying on bed. If chest sinks into mattress, immediately place on firm surface, for example a floor or place a large tray under child.
- Compress heart repeatedly while lung inflation is being carried out. The force of compression should depress the chest by one third of the antero-posterior diameter.

D. Diagnosis / Disease / Drugs

- When more staff arrive, the most experienced continues resuscitation while the others assist.
- Try to define the cause of the collapse.
- Start an IV infusion if possible.

Task of the assistant:
- Connect oxygen.
- Fetch and connect suction.

- Cardiac massage.
- If no IV already running, then assemble:
  - Small bottle / bag IV fluid, for example Saline or Darrows.
  - Drip set and IV cannula or scalp vein set.
  - Strapping.
  - 20 ml syringe and 15 needle.
  - 2 ml syringe.
  - Have 50% dextrose, 8,5% sodium bicarbonate, and adrenaline available.
- An intraosseous puncture may be needed if an intravenous line cannot be established.
- Do not leave patient unless you are told to do so.

Drowning (Or near drowning)

More commonly found in one to four year age group. The main problems of near-drowning are hypoxaemia, water inhalation, and hypothermia.

Hypoxaemia due to submersion results in:
- Ineffective circulation after about three minutes.
- Irreversible cerebral changes after about five minutes (altered by temperature of water).
- Severe acidosis.
- Submersion in very cold water may result in hypothermia (body temperature below 30 °C).
- About 10% of victims die acutely of laryngospasm, but this may also protect against inhalation of water as long as effective resuscitation is then carried out.

Prevention
- Enclose pools and exercise caution at dams, rivers, and beaches.
- Remember toddlers can drown in half-full buckets or drums.

Treatment
- Immediate ventilation, oxygenation, and circulatory support are critical.
- The effective resuscitation of the near-drowned patient during the acute phase is the most important single factor governing recovery.
- All patients with a history of significant submersion, even though asymptomatic, should be admitted to hospital for at least 24 hours

because of the risk of late development of pulmonary oedema.
- Rewarming is an urgent matter in hypothermia. Consciousness is lost at a core temperature below 30 °C.
- Rewarm in a bath at 40–44 °C.
- IV administration of sodium bicarbonate may be indicated.

Complications
- Death / cerebral damage and cerebral oedema.
- Pulmonary oedema which may be acute or delayed.
- Bacterial pneumonia and aspiration of vomitus, dirty water.
- Atelectasis and pneumothorax.

Electrocutions
Electrical injuries and electrocution result from domestic electricity and lightning. Passage of electricity through the body causes local heating and skin burns, often with marked underlying necrosis. Internal injury may also result.

Death results from
- Hypoxia due to electrically induced tetanic contractions of the chest wall.
- Cardiac arrhythmias such as ventricular fibrillation or cardiac asystole.
- Gross tissue disruptions in death from lightning.
- Severe burns.

Symptoms
- Severe collapse (shock).
- Unconsciousness.
- Severe pain from skin burns.
- Pain from muscular injuries or dislocations of joints (from severe muscular contractions).
- Faintness and anxiety.
- Retrograde amnesia.

Prevention
- Need for safe design of installations of electrical circuits with circuit breakers.
- Proper earthing of all electrical equipment.

Treatment
- Remove the person in contact with electrical conductor safely:

  - ○ Switch off the current if possible.
  - ○ Use an insulated pole to dislodge the patient from the electricity.
  - ○ Stand on dry rubber mat or wear dry rubber boots.
  - ○ Hold on to the clothes of victim rather than the body.
- If unconscious, start resuscitation.
- Examine for burns and treat.
- Examine for fractures.
- Refer to hospital.

Poisoning

Always try to obtain the original container of fluid or tablets taken. Try to find out how many tablets or how much of the liquid was taken and when the substance was taken. Use direct Poison Line to nearest referral hospital for advice on specific management.

Poisoning or drug overdosage may be a manifestation of child abuse. Remember the child may have accompanying illness with symptoms other than those resulting from the ingestion of the drug or poison.

Interpretation of signs and symptoms (<u>Need to check with poison centre</u>)

Excitement, hallucinations
Belladonna group
Tranquillisers
Alcohol
Phenothiazines

Confusion
Tranquillisers

Coma
Alcohol
Anti-convulsants

Convulsions
Turpentine

Spasms
Phenothiazines
Anti-epilepsy drugs
Solvent sniffing

Dilated pupils
Barbiturates
Amphetamines

Dry mouth
Belladonna group
Amphetamines

Salivation
Organophosphate
Insecticides

Ataxia
Alcohol

Bradycardia
Digoxin
Lily of the Valley

Small pupils
Opiates
Organophosphate
Insecticides
Phenothiazines

Tachycardia
Alcohol

**Burns in and around
the mouth**
Caustics
Acids or alkalis

Specific antidotes for toxic substances found in the home exist in only a very small percentage of cases, for example Narcan® in opiate overdose.

General management of any poisoning
- Universal antidote, for example milk.
- Gastric aspiration and washout with saline if the toxic substance was ingested within six hours. Do not attempt to empty the stomach in paraffin or petrol ingestion, or ingestion of strong acids or alkalis.
- Activated charcoal 1 g/kg in 100 ml water can be given after gastric emptying.
- Maintain vital functions during transfer, that is, respiratory and cardiac function.
- Administer specific antidote if known and available (seldom the case).
- Take blood sample for toxicology screen.

Common forms of poisoning
- **Paraffin**: Avoid vomiting. Start antibiotics.
- **Salicylate**: Manage with gastric emptying, rehydration, forced alkaline diuresis if possible.
- **Organophosphate**: Wash the patient thoroughly, remove all old clothing and give intravenous atropine repeatedly until the pupils are mid-point dilated.
- **Barbiturates**: Treat with gastric emptying, intravenous fluids to increase diuresis and maintain respiration at all costs.
- **Iron**: Treat with gastric emptying, put bicarbonate solution into stomach. Empty bowel with Go-lytely®. May require desferrioxamine.

Milk can be used at home as a universal antidote. However, this must not be given if there is a depressed level of consciousness, as the child may vomit and aspirate. In hospitals, activated charcoal is used as a universal antidote.
Get the patient transferred to hospital as soon as possible.

Poisonous bites and stings

Bee and wasp stings

These cause pain, with vascular and tissue damage which is usually confined to the affected area. In hypersensitive persons, one sting can cause a fatal anaphylactic reaction. In rare instances, the site of the sting is dangerous due to the effects of acute oedema, for example in the tongue or throat.

Treatment of bee or wasp stings

- With bee stings, wipe away the remaining sting with edge of blunt knife (do not pinch with tweezers or fingers).
- Wasps don't leave their stings behind.
- Ice water or an ice cube may relieve the local pain.
- If anaphylactic symptoms, antihistamine and adrenaline 1:1 000 by injection (see section on anaphylaxis). Refer urgently to hospital.
- If bronchospasm present, give a bronchodilator.

Bluebottle sting

- Pull (don't rub) off tentacles still adherent.
- Sodium bicarbonate paste (baking soda). Apply and leave on sting.
- Apply meat tenderiser or vinegar.
- If neither are available, rub with sea sand or talcum powder after removing tentacles.

Scorpion sting

This normally produces only local pain, but in a small child the sting may cause death. Scorpions with big tails and small pincers are the most poisonous. They do not bite. Their sting is at the tip of the tail.

Treatment of scorpion stings

- In a child over five years who appears generally well and who has local pain only, give paracetamol, local ice packs, and observe. Local anaesthetic is effective for pain.
- All children of five and under, or any child who becomes ill with weakness, drowsiness or vomiting, should be referred to hospital immediately.

Snake bites

Most snakes are not poisonous, and poison may not be injected when a person is bitten. The type of poison and the effects on the patient depend on the species of snake and size and health of the victim.

Nature of poison
  Adders: The venom causes local death of tissue, leading to severe local pain and swelling.
  Cobras and mambas: Muscle paralysis with respiratory and cardiac difficulties within half to six hours.
  Boomslang (rare): Severe generalised bleeding tendency after 48 hours.

Management
- Look for fang marks to make sure that the child has been bitten.
- If the snake was killed, it should be brought to the hospital for identification if possible.
- Most snake bites are caused by the puffadder. This is a fat, brown snake with yellow stripes and spots with a triangular shaped head. Do not use a tourniquet, but reassure the patient and transfer to hospital immediately. Do not give antivenom unless child under two years or delay in transfer.
- In definite cobra or mamba bites, use a tight compression bandage and give snake bite antiserum (both ampoules) intravenously or IM proximal to the bite before urgent transfer to hospital. Give oxygen and mouth-to-mouth ventilation if needed. Patients may be serum-sensitive if any previous horse serum injection has been administered. Be ready to treat anaphylaxis with adrenaline.
- Cutting or sucking the wound or using local medicines are useless. If a snake spits into a patient's eyes, the poison causes severe pain and redness. Wash out repeatedly with water or diluted antiserum and refer to hospital.

Application of a broad compression bandage tourniquet:
Pressure should be similar to that when binding a sprained ankle. The bandage must not be used as a tourniquet. Bandage the whole limb if possible. Only use a torniquet for a definite cobra or mumba bite if antivenum will not be available for several hours.

Spider bites
This usually causes only local pain and redness. An abscess may develop after a few days. Death is extremely uncommon except in button spider bites in young children. Button spider bites cause severe abdominal pain and shock and may need antiserum treatment.

Management

- Panado® and ice packs for pain.
- Penicillin if the bite appears to be infected.
- Refer to hospital if the child becomes ill, for example pyrexial, shocked, drowsy, weak or vomits.

Procedures and techniques

Restraining the patient

Restraint is necessary in almost every procedure. The age and compliance of the child are the key factors influencing the choice of method. Preparation of the patient includes optimal restraint through human holding and 'wrapping' techniques. Exposure of the procedure site, adequate lighting, and a comfortable position for the 'operator' are important for success. Sedation is often not administered as it takes time to work. It then becomes more difficult to apply adequate restraint, and haste may well result in wasting time.

Methods of restraint
- Wrapping the whole body and pinning it in a sheet.
- Physical restraint: Patient is held in the optimal position by an experienced helper, for example a nurse for lumbar puncture.
- Splinting of limb.
- Restraining to the bed with arm and / or leg tie-downs.
- Restrains of the patient to prevent IV lines, drains, etc. being pulled out.
- Sedation, analgesia, and local anaesthesia.

Note: It is usually safe and helpful to administer either sedation or analgesia or both. Consider the patient's physical condition and the underlying disease process when deciding on the form and dosage of required medications.

Taking blood

General principles
- Decide on which tests are important for diagnosis and management.
- Get consent for procedure required.
- Make arrangements with laboratory (if necessary) for specimens to be examined.
- Obtain maximum data from taking blood once only.
- Select proper equipment.

- Collect the required amount and type of blood sample for the test. Use the correct tubes.
- Inform and comfort the patient and parents.
- Label and deliver blood specimens promptly before they deteriorate.

Sources of blood
- Venous, arterial, and capillary.

Equipment
- Gloves (HIV).
- Sterile disposable syringes.
- Needle or scalp vein set.
- Tourniquet / baumanometer.
- Specimen containers.
- Antiseptics: Alcohol swabs or sterile swabs with Hibicol®.
- Strapping.
- Laboratory forms as required.
- Experienced assistant to restrain the child.
- Sedation, if required, must be adequate and properly timed.

Procedures
- Identify child.
- Take child to procedure room.
- Wash hands and wear gloves.
- Position child as required with an experienced person holding and restraining the child.

Venipuncture
- This is a done by placing a hypodermic needle through the skin into a vein.
- Needle attached to syringe.
- Use scalp vein set in small infants.

Selection of site
- Veins of forearm and antecubital fossa.
  - Site of choice for children 2–3 years, because veins are superficial, easily visible, and palpable.
  - In older child, vein may only be palpable.
  - Common sources of difficulty:
    - Incorrect position.
    - Inadequate restraint.

- Needle with too long a bevel (goes through vein).
- Collapse of vein (aspiration too forceful).
- Use of alcohol sponge on puncture site (painful).
- Hazards:
  - Infection: Cellulitis, abscess, osteomyelitis.
  - Haematoma.
  - Failure to remove tourniquet: Ischemia.
  - Viral hepatitis from contaminated equipment, syringes, and needles.
  - Arterial trauma: An aberrant artery in antecubital area, found in 10% of the population. Because of close proximity, could be mistaken for vein. Bright red blood should raise suspicion.
  - Needle prick to nurse / doctor: Hepatitis B, HIV risk.
- External jugular vein – position and restraint:
  - Infant placed in supine position and body restraint applied.
  - Head and neck suspended off edge of table and held in hands of assistant.
  - Shoulders firmly on table.
  - Head turned 45–60° to one side of midline.
  - Child should be crying to distend the veins.
  - Difficult and not recommended in very young infants.
- Veins on dorsum of hand and foot.
- Scalp veins:
  - Shave hair first. Use only as last alternative.
- Posterior fontanelle, internal jugular, and femoral vein: To be used in emergencies by doctors only. Potentially dangerous.

Capillary puncture

- Equipment: Disposable lancet, Vaseline®.
- Sites:
  - Heel puncture (neonate).
  - Finger puncture (child over two years: index, middle or ring).
  - Ear lobe.
  - Big toe (medial aspect).
- First warm site from which blood is to be taken.
- A thin layer of Vaseline® on the skin (especially heel in neonates) helps form a 'bead' of blood.
- Common sources of error in capillary puncture:
  - Insufficient depth of incision.
  - Dull or barbed lancet.
  - Blood from oedematous, cold, vasoconstricted or cyanotic part.

- ○ Puncture through wet film or antiseptic: May produce haemolysis and prevent formation of rounded 'bead' of blood at site of puncture, making collection difficult.
- ○ Excessive squeezing in immediate neighbourhood of puncture will produce dilution of blood specimen and favour clotting.
- ○ Use of incorrect lancet: A round puncture instrument such as a hypodermic needle or stylet will not induce a free flow of blood.

Record procedure, type of investigations, and date sent in folder.

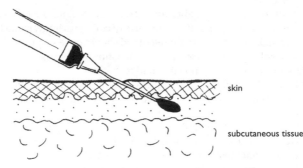

Figure A.1 Intradermal injection

Preparations given by injection

Intradermal (Into the skin)
- For example PPD (Mantoux test for tuberculosis).
- Sites: Ventral (inner) surface of the left forearm.

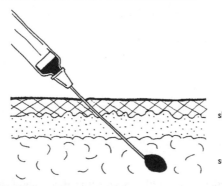

Figure A.2 Subcutaneous injection

Hypodermic or subcutaneous *(Into the loose tissue spaces just beneath the skin)*
- For example insulin.
- Sites: Any site on limb or trunk where loose tissue space under the skin is obvious. Rotate site when repeated injections given, for example insulin in diabetics.

Intramuscular *(IM)*
- The needle is inserted at right angles to the skin and care is taken to ensure that the needle has not entered a vein or artery by slightly withdrawing the plunger before giving the injection. If blood appears in syringe, withdraw and inject elsewhere.
- Sites:
  o Thigh (quadriceps) muscle mass of the outer third of the thigh. In general, the only permissible site for intramuscular injections in neonates and young children. Avoid anteromedial area which contains vital structures such as the femoral vein, artery, and nerve.

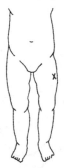

Figure A.3 Quadriceps muscle injection

  o Upper outer quadrant of the buttocks: Use only if given specific written instructions. Nerve on inner lower side or sciatic nerve may be damaged. Not recommended in children.
  o Deltoid muscle in the lateral aspect of the upper arm: Not generally used except for measles vaccine 0,5 ml, tetanus toxoid 0,5 ml, and pertussis 0,5 ml. (These may also be administered subcutaneously.) This site may be used in other instances if no other site is available, for example in burns. Total volume must never exceed 1 ml.

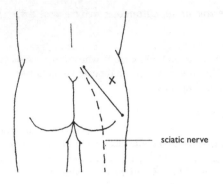

Figure A.4 Buttock injection

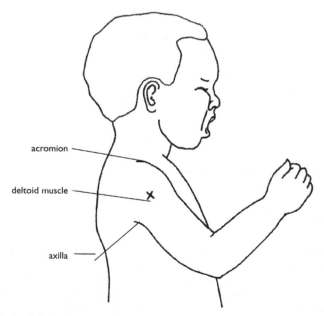

Figure A.5 Deltoid injection

- Volume determined by weight and muscle bulk rather than age.
  - Up to 2,5 kg: Maximum 0,5 ml per site.
  - 2,5–5 kg: Maximum 1 ml per site.
  - 5–10 kg: Maximum 1,5 ml per site.
  - Over 10 kg: Maximum 2,0 ml per site.
- The nature of the substance should be taken into consideration, for example Bicillin LA® (thick substances) not more than 1 ml per site in children under three years.
- General comments:
  - Identify patient, medication, and dosage.
  - The infant or child must be restrained by a second person to assure safe and correct administration.
  - Sites should be rotated if injection is to be repeated. Keep a record of these sites.
  - IM injections, particularly Paraldehyde®, should be given deep into the muscle to prevent abscess formation.
  - Glass syringes should ideally be used for Paraldehyde®. Plastic syringes may be used in an emergency if a glass syringe is not available, provided the injection is administered immediately after the Paraldehyde® is drawn into the syringe. If left for any time, Paraldehyde® dissolves plastic.
  - Correct needles must be used for intramuscular injections: Size 26 for neonates and size 22 for other children are recommended.
  - All needles, lancets, etc. must be disposed of in a 'sharps' container to prevent accidental pricks to anyone, not only the person doing the procedure.

Intravenous (IV)

IV therapy is hazardous and must not be taken lightly or given indiscriminately.

- Precautions and possible hazards:
  - Careful use of sterile needle / scalp vein set.
  - Check that giving set is not faulty.
  - Check correct fluid is given to correct child.
  - Inspect container and contents, see that it is not leaking and fluid in it is not cloudy.
  - Change giving sets every 24 hours.
  - All fluid to be documented on patient's chart.
  - Check additives given into bag, drip chamber or bulb.
  - Label accurately if any additives to bag / bottle.

- Take care when applying splints: Not too tight or pressure necrosis may result.
- Take care that injection is not into an artery (bright red blood), as necrosis may follow.
- In either of last two instances, the result may be sloughing of tissue and severe scarring.
- Do not allow infusion to run in too fast, as rapid injection of some substances can have fatal results. For example, potassium given too quickly may give rise to ventricular fibrillation, and calcium may produce bradycardia followed by cardiac arrest.
- Use only a drip controller and not a pump for all hyperosmolar / irritative fluids.
- Accessible superficial veins:
  - Scalp, especially infants.
  - Back of hand.
  - Arm, cephalic / basilic veins in antecubital fossa.
  - Forearm.
  - Ankle.
  - Foot.
  - Neck (external jugular).
  - Umbilicus (neonates).
- Scalp veins
  - Advantages:
    - Only arms need be restrained.
    - Usually the most accessible in infants.
    - Infiltration of tissue outside vein can be easily seen.
    - Needle can be firmly strapped.
    - Several vessels available in the same area.
  - Disadvantages:
    - Often upsetting to parents.
    - May be necessary to shave hair, which takes a long time to grow.
    - Infections may result, such as scalp abscess, or intracranial venous sinus, pericranium or brain sepsis.

Methods of venipuncture

- If anatomic site permits, occlude using tourniquet (baumanometer cuff) or another nurse's hands.
- Clean skin with antiseptic (don't touch site thereafter).
- Shave hair if necessary (after parent's consent obtained).
- Check needle to see if point sharp and not hooked or blunt.
- Run fluid through IV set and scalp vein needle.

- Stretch skin and anchor vein with thumb or index finger of free hand.
- Insert needle.
- When blood flows back into tubing, remove tourniquet or other constricting appliance and open clamp on IV tubing.
- Attach needle securely to skin.
- Regulate the speed of drip.

General remarks
- Right-handed children prefer infusion in left arm.
- Avoid using a vein near a joint. Movement may dislodge needle.
- Methods of distending a vein:
  - Apply baumanometer cuff or rubber band. Gradually release until arterial pulse palpable. Then maintain pressure at this level until needle in vein. Release pressure completely.
  - Rubber band around scalp.
  - Open and close hand, keep hand tightly closed until vein entered.
  - By vasodilation: Place hand or foot in warm water to distend veins.

Intraspinal (Into spinal cord)
- Level 3 or 4 lumbar spinous interspace.
- To be done by doctors with training only.

Lumbar puncture

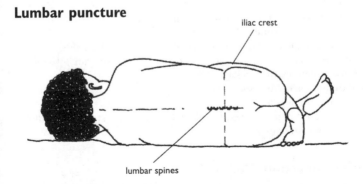

Figure A.6 Lumbar puncture

Proper position and restraint is critical for a successful tap. Neonates and small infants are often punctured in the sitting position when the head and neck are not flexed. The lateral recumbent position is employed in older infants and children. Shoulders and hips should be at right angles to the bed or table. The operator's line of vision should be on the same horizontal as the puncture site. The lumbar spine must be flexed, but avoid pressure flexion of the neck while attempting to flex the back. Put pressure on shoulders rather than the head and neck. Ensure that all apparatus, for example needles, stylets, manometers, tubes, are available.

The site of the puncture is the interspace between L3–4 or L4–5. A line joining the highest points of two iliac crests passes just above the fourth lumbar spine. (See Figure A.6.) After anaesthetising skin and tissue down to the laminae, insert the short bevelled needle with stylet in the midline between L3–L4. The bevel should be in the long axis of the dura so as to part the fibres and not cut across them. Loss of resistance is felt as the needle penetrates the ligamentum flavum. The next 'pop' occurs as the needle penetrates the dura. Remove the stylet and if no fluid emerges, turn the needle through 90°. If the tap is dry, replace the stylet and advance the needle a little further. Check as before for fluid. The distance between the skin and subarachnoid space is 1,5–2,5 cm in infants; 5 cm in three- to five-year olds, and 6–8 cm in adolescents. Pressure should be measured with a manometer in all non-crying and non-struggling patients. Normal pressure is 60–160 mm CSF.

Dangers
- Coning may occur immediately or after a few hours due to ongoing leakage of spinal fluid.
- Any indication of raised intracranial pressure, especially altered level of consciousness, is a contraindication to lumbar puncture. Absence of papilloedema is not a reliable sign.
- Introduction of infection.
- Breakage of needle.
- Introduction of dermis resulting in a dermoid (non-styletted needle).
- Nerve or cord damage.

Urine collection (Methods)

Collection bag
Clean external genitalia with soap and water, and dry with sterile swabs. Apply a disposable sterile plastic bag with a non-irritating adhesive cover over the penis or onto the perineum. Leave exposed for observation. Collect sample immediately after passing. Bag samples are often

contaminated. Negative cultures exclude a urinary tract infection. This method is widely used for obtaining 'routine' specimens in the infant.

'Clean catch' with voluntary voiding

Method can be used in children over three years of age. Very unsatisfactory in infants. Glans (and foreskin if present) or perineum must be thoroughly cleaned with soap and water and / or an antiseptic and dried. A midstream catch is then collected during voiding with the foreskin drawn back or labia held apart.

Bladder catheterisation

Potentially hazardous; the specimen must be important enough to warrant the procedure. Single-specimen catheterisation is safer than an indwelling catheter. The procedure must be done under sterile conditions with gloves, careful cleaning (see above), and with foreskin drawn back or labia held apart. A lubricated thin catheter or F8 feeding tube is passed directly into the urethral meatus and advanced gently until urine specimen is obtained into a sterile tube. The catheter is then carefully removed.

Suprapubic needle aspiration

Indicated if urinalysis is urgent, the perineum excoriated, or a previous culture was of doubtful significance in a child under the age of two years.

The full bladder is found intra-abdominally by percussion and is therefore accessible. Change and feed the baby. After 30 minutes, check whether the nappy is still dry and the bladder full. The baby is then placed supine and immobilised in a frog position by an assistant. The lower abdomen is cleaned. The aspiration site is located in the midline 1–2 cm above the symphysis pubis. The needle and syringe are held 10–20° from perpendicular to the abdominal wall pointing towards the pelvis. The needle is advanced through the abdominal wall with gentle aspiration on the syringe. Bladder entry occurs 1–2,5 cm of advancement. If no urine is obtained, attempt a second time with a further 10–15° angulation, aiming more into the pelvis. If still dry, cease further attempts. When cleaning the abdomen, be prepared for a midstream 'catch' specimen, as urine is often voided at this stage of the proceedings.

Dangers
- Introduction of infection.
- Local haematoma.
- Bowel perforation and peritonitis.

Nasogastric tube

- Passing a nasogastric tube may be done for the following reasons:
  - To instill a milk formula, electrolyte solution, or medications.
  - To remove the gastric contents (toxin / poison).
  - To remove amniotic fluid in neonate.
  - To obtain diagnostic material, for example for the diagnosis of tuberculosis or for post-operative decompression.

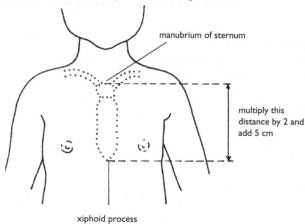

manubrium of sternum

multiply this distance by 2 and add 5 cm

xiphoid process

Figure A.7 Nasogastric tube length

- If the child is old enough, explain what is going to be done. Perform the procedure when the patient is sitting with his or her back firmly supported. In the younger child or infant, place in supine position with bodily restraint and an assistant to help.
- Select the appropriate tube. Measure length to be passed by measuring the distance from manubrium sterni to xiphisternum. Double this and add 5 cm for feeding, aspiration, and / or drainage. Mark the tube at the selected length. Lubricate first 3–4 cm with KY jelly or water. With head slightly flexed, pass the tube through the nostril aiming for the occiput (not vertex). If resistance is encountered, withdraw, and try again. If still unsuccessful, try the other side. Ask the patient to try to make swallowing motions despite gagging. Continue to pass the tube to the selected length. If severe coughing, choking or colour change occurs, withdraw immediately. Fix the tube lightly to the cheek and

aspirate with a syringe. Test with litmus (blue turns pink if acid). If no fluid is aspirated, advance 3 cm and try again. If still no fluid is aspirated and you are sure the tube is in the stomach, instill 3 ml of 0,9% saline. If there is any coughing, spluttering or cyanosis, withdraw the tube immediately. Replace. Alternatively, place the bell of your stethoscope over the stomach area. Inject 5–10 ml of air rapidly down the tube. A gurgling noise on auscultation indicates that the tip of the tube is in the stomach. Less reliable method in newborns. Restrain as necessary and fix tube firmly to cheek using wrap-around and V-strapping.

Dangers

- Vomiting with aspiration while doing the procedure.
- Ulceration or infection of nasal mucosa or epistaxis.
- Placement of the tube in tracheobronchial tree.
- Otitis media or sinusitis with prolonged use.
- Coiling or knotting of tube with inability to remove it.

Intraosseous infusion route *(For life-saving fluid administration)*

In an emergency, for example shock, where several attempts to place an IV line have failed, use the intraosseous route. The most suitable site is 2 cm below the tibial tuberosity. A wide-bore needle (15–18 gauge) can be used if a needle with stylet is not available. In children under 18 months, an 18 x 1.5 or 20 x 1.5 lumbar puncture needle is suitable. Hold the needle perpendicular to the skin and, with a twisting movement, push it into the flat part of the tibia until a 'give' is felt. The needle is now in the bone marrow cavity. Do not advance it further. In a shocked patient, fluid must be introduced under pressure (use a 20 ml syringe as a 'push-in' or a sphygmomanometer cuff wrapped around a collapsible IV plastic fluid container). The dosage and volume of drugs and fluid are the same as for direct IV infusion (see p. 171).

Protocols of management for some common conditions

Common conditions

Anaemia
Asthma
 ○ Mild
 ○ Moderate to severe
Burns
Conjunctivitis
Convulsions
Diarrhoea (acute)
Diarrhoea (chronic)
Head lice
Herpes stomatitis
Impetigo
Kwashiorkor
Infectious hepatitis
Measles
Meningococcal infection
Neonatal problems
 ○ Convulsions
 ○ Haemorrhagic disease
 ○ Jaundice
 ○ Umbilical sepsis
Nephritis

Otitis media
Otorrhoea
Parasites
 ○ Ascariasis
 ○ Pinworm
 ○ Trichuris
Pneumonia
Poisoning: general
  measures
Rheumatic fever
Ringworm
 ○ Body
 ○ Scalp
Scabies
Shock
Stridor
Squint
Trauma
 ○ Lacerations
 ○ Fractures
Whooping cough

In all cases, explain the nature and likely course of the illness to parents or guardians, as well as what complications to look out for, and what to do should they occur.

In some areas, the recommended action may not yet be legally carried out by nurses. In these cases, a doctor must be consulted for authorisation of such actions. These include the use or issue of certain medications (those falling within Schedule 4 and up), and the ordering of certain investigations, such as X-rays.

The word 'refer' used in the following pages means refer to a doctor or transfer to hospital.

ACTION

REFER

Anaemia (See p. 180)

- Look for underlying cause.
- Ferrous sulphate syrup (continue for one month after haemoglobin back to normal level).
- Vermox®: One tablet twice daily for three days.
- Advise on iron-containing green vegetables, liver, and eggs in diet.
- Stress importance of continuing iron medication for a long period.
- Mention that stools may change to a grey or black colour while on iron.
- Check haemoglobin after two weeks.

- No haemoglobin rise after two weeks of therapy.
- Purpura.
- Enlargement of liver or spleen.
- Haematuria.
- Haemoglobin under 7,5 g/100 ml.

Asthma (See p. 281)

Mild

- Salbutamol (Ventolin®) or fenoteral (Berotec®) aerosol pump (metered inhaler) with spacer if possible; two puffs to relieve wheezing.

Moderate to severe

- Salbutamol or fenoterol 0,5 ml in 1 ml saline by nebulisation (may be repeated after 30 minutes).
- Treat any bacterial infection with amoxicillin.
- Encourage fluid intake.
- Reassure patient.
- Oxygen as needed.

- Insufficient relief of wheezing after second nebulisation.

ACTION	REFER

Burns (See p. 318)

- Treat shock if present. Ensure good fluid intake or IV.
- Paracetamol for pain.
- Tetanus toxoid.
- Dressing / Povidone iodine 5% cream.
- Keep burned area clean.
- Assess urinary output; this must be maintained.
- Regular dressings.

- If 5% or more of body surface involved, or if there is associated shock.
- If any sign of infection.
- Involvement of face, perineum, hands, feet, flexures.
- Circumferential wounds with loss of skin elasticity.
- Electrical burns.

Conjunctivitis (See p. 252)

- Eye swabs to laboratory.
- Clean eye with preboiled water or saline irrigation.
- Antibiotic eye ointment e.g. chloromycetin, erythromycin.
- See again in three days, or sooner if condition worsens.

- Neonates with persistent conjunctivitis or cellulitis.
- Persistent discharge despite treatment.
- Suspected blocked lacrimal duct.

Convulsions (See p. 130)

- Rectal diazepam (Valium®) 0,5 mg/kg (maximum 10 mg).
- Clear air passages.
- Insert airway if necessary.
- Anti-fever measures.
- Reagent strips. If low glucose, give 2 ml/kg of 50% dextrose water by nasogastric tube or 1–2 ml/kg by IV infusion (maximum 10 ml).

- All neonates (urgently).
- All other cases after emergency treatment.
- Known epileptics (not urgent), to improve medication and control.

ACTION	REFER

ACTION

- Check BP, urine for blood / protein.
- Check for neck stiffness.

Diarrhoea (Acute) (See p. 161)
Not dehydrated and not vomiting

- Stop solids but continue breast- or bottle feeds.
- Give additional oral glucose / electrolyte solution ('ORS'); as much as child will take.
- Educate parents in bottle and feeding hygiene. See patient again as soon as possible, at least by next day.

Not dehydrated but vomiting

- Stop milk feeds.
- Give glucose / electrolyte solution ('ORS') while under observation (for 12 hours) orally or by continuous intragastric drip.
- Start IV fluids if patient becomes dehydrated despite above 'ORS' treatment.

Dehydrated (See p. 162)

- IV or Intragastric fluids (see Fluid therapy, pp. 168–174).

Diarrhoea (Chronic)

- Stool for microscopy culture and sensitivity.

REFER

- If vomiting persists.
- If child becomes listless or drowsy.
- Start IV fluids before transfer (or intragastric drip).

- All cases who remain shocked.
- Before transfer, treat shock with IV fluids or intragastric drip if IV not possible.

- No response to Flagyl®.
- Failure to thrive.

ACTION

- Test for lactose intolerance. If positive, give lactose-free milk, e.g. soya milk, for two weeks; then try full cream milk again.
- If above test is negative, try a course of metronidazole (Flagyl®).
- Parents to monitor child's hygiene to prevent parasitic infestation, e.g. child to wash hands before meals, etc.

Head lice (See p. 294)

- 1% gamma benzene hexachloride (lotion or shampoo); apply to entire scalp and leave for five minutes.
- Wash hair with soap or shampoo.
- Comb hair with nit comb (fine comb). Very curly hair is difficult to comb with nit comb. May be necessary to cut hair short or shave scalp. Parents' permission required for this.
- Repeat one week later.
- Explain condition is contagious.
- Parents to report child's condition to school principal.

REFER

- Blood or mucus in stool.
- Pale (fatty) smelly stools (query malabsorption).

ACTION	REFER

Herpes stomatitis (See p. 140)

- Keep mouth clean with mouth wash, e.g. glycothymol or sodiuo bicarbonate.
- Paracetamol.
- Encourage fluid intake.
- IV or intragastric fluid (if dehydrated) prior to referral.

REFER
- Dehydration (refusing oral fluids).
- Extensive spread.
- Complications, e.g. drowsiness, hepatomegaly, stridor.

Impetigo

- Soak to remove crusts. Wash with Savlon® or Betadine® lotion.
- Vioform in zinc ointment to body lesions.
- Vioform in emulsifying ointment for head, both three times daily for about seven days.
- Treat accompanying scabies and lice if present.
- If severe or extensive, oral amoxicillin or erythromycin for five to ten days.
- Daily washing helps prevent infection.
- Emphasise infectious nature.
- Explain role of biting insects (e.g. fleas) in causing condition.

REFER
- Failure to respond to treatment.
- Complications: glomerulonephritis.

Kwashiorkor (See p. 62)

- Treat infection with co-trimoxazole.

REFER
- All cases of kwashiorkor should ideally be admitted to hospital, as it is a life-threatening condition.

ACTION

- Feed milk 120 mg/kg/day. Frequent feeds of small volume.
- Introduce solids, e.g. mince / beans / stew, when feeds well tolerated.
- Oral potassium chloride 0,5 g eight-hourly for three days.
- Vermox® / Zentel®.
- Flagyl® (five days).
- Iron therapy only after oedema has subsided.
- See patient weekly for some time.
- Educate parents on nutrition and need for regular follow-up.
- Investigate social situation.

Infectious hepatitis (See p. 205)
- No specific measures.
- Diet. What the child wants. Small nutritious meals, plenty of fluids.
- Emphasise faecal / oral risk of spread.
- Rest at home, not necessarily in bed.
- Notify local authority.
- The child usually starts to feel better after jaundice appears and improves further about seven days after the onset. Duration of jaundice is variable. Urine may remain dark for several weeks.

REFER

- Excess vomiting.
- Signs of liver failure: drowsy, tremor, ataxia.
- Signs of chronic liver disease:
  - Clubbing, oedema.
  - Hard liver or spleen.
  - Ascites.
- Jaundice not fading by two weeks.

ACTION

Measles (See p. 214)
- Anti-fever measures.
- Vitamin A 200 000 IU orally on two successive days.
- Antibiotic, e.g. amoxicillin for seven days.
- Eye ointment, if painful eyes.
- Encourage fluids.
- Tepid sponge if high fever.
- Watch for complications, e.g. rapid breathing.
- Notify health authorities.

Meningococcal infection
(See p. 217)
- Treat shock, if present.
- Blood culture, if possible.
- Start IV penicillin urgently.
- Treat contacts with Rifampicin®.

Neonatal problems
Convulsions (See p. 130)
- Stop convulsion with phenobarbitone 10 mg/kg IM.
- Maintain airway.
- Give oxygen if cyanosed.
- Check blood glucose concentration.

Haemorrhagic disease of
newborn (See p. 102)
- Give vitamin K1 (Konakion®) 1 mg IM (IV if possible).
- Check PCV or haemoglobin level.
- IV therapy if required (shock).

REFER

- If dehydrated.
- Pneumonia is not responding to therapy.
- Any other complications not responding.
- For X-ray if necessary (chest symptoms).
- Associated herpes stomatitis.

- All cases as soon as condition is stabilised.

- All cases.

- All cases.

ACTION

- May need a blood transfusion.

Jaundice *(See p. 103)*
- Measure TSB if possible.
- Phototherapy if indicated (see chart).
- Look for possible source of infection.

Umbilical sepsis *(See p. 106)*
- Clean umbilical stump with spirits three-hourly.

Nephritis (See p. 273)
- Test urine, check haemoglobin, weight, and blood pressure.
- Take throat swab.
- X-ray chest if possible.
- Blood to be taken for chemistry: urea, creatinine, electrolytes, serum complement, protein ASOT, full blood count if laboratory service available.
- Penicillin V or amoxicillin for ten days.
- Fluid, protein, salt restriction.
- Measure urine output.
- Bed rest.
- See daily for urine and BP check until improving.

REFER

- All cases of severe jaundice.
- All infants who are clinically sick.

- If any abdominal wall oedema or signs of septicaemia. Give antibiotic and refer.

- All cases should be referred to hospital.

ACTION

Otitis media (Acute) (See p. 149)
- Amoxicillin or
  co-trimoxazole for ten days.
- Antipyretic, e.g.
  paracetamol.
- Decongestant, e.g.
  Iliadin®, Otrivin® or Demazin®
  nose drops for three days.
- See next day and at intervals
  thereafter.
- After an attack of acute
  otitis media, ear drum
  may not return to normal
  for two to three weeks.

Otorrhoea (See p. 151)
(Persistent discharge from ears)
- Medications as for acute
  otitis media (above).
- Anti-fever measures, if
  needed.
- Decongestant, as for
  acute otitis.
- At first visit, carefully
  clean / clear ear canal with
  cotton
  wool on orange stick
  (dry mopping).
  Exclude foreign body.
- Boric acid (antiseptic)
  ear drops.
- Demonstrate method and
  instruct parents to clean
  ears night and morning.
- See within seven to ten days.

REFER

- Not responding after
  course of antibiotics.
- Discharging ear not
  drying up.
- Repeated infections.
- Pain persists despite
  treatment.

- No response to two
  courses of antibiotics.
- High posterior, or central
  perforations which
  do not close after two to three
  months of observation.
- Presence of anterior or

  attic perforation.
- Any pain, tenderness or
  swelling in the mastoid
  area.

ACTION	REFER

Parasites

Pinworm (Enterobius) *(See p. 263)*

- Albendazole (Zentel®): Under 2 years: 200 mg single dose. Older than 2 years: 400 mg single dose. or
- Mebendazole (Vermox®) one tablet or 5 ml twice daily for three days.
- Parents to bath child regularly, cut nails short, prevent scratching.

- No response to two courses of treatment.

Roundworm (Ascaris)
(See p. 264)

- Vermox®: One tablet twice daily for three days (more expensive); or
- Zentel®: Under 2 years: 200 mg single dose. Older than 2 years: 400 mg single dose.
- Advice to parents: Child to wash hands before eating, wash vegetables, avoid eating dirt, good faecal disposal, treat all children in household at risk.

Whipworm (Trichuris)
(See p. 268)

- Mebendazole (Vermox®) one tablet twice daily for three days; or
- Zentel®: Under 2 years: 200 mg single dose. Older than 2 years: 400 mg single dose.
- Assess nutrition. Improving diet reduces worm load.

ACTION	REFER

- Parents to assist in preventing reinfestation by washing child's hands before eating, washing vegetables, good faecal disposal, prevention of dirt-eating.

Pneumonia (See p. 285)
- Anti-fever measures.
- Oral amoxicillin, co-trimoxazole or erythromycin.
- If cyanosed, give oxygen by face mask while awaiting transfer.
- If not cleared by tenth day, do Mantoux test or refer.
- See daily if possible.

REFER
- Breathing faster than 60/minute.
- Recession.
- Alar flare.
- Cyanosis.
- Drowsiness.
- Confusion.
- Not improving on treatment.

Poisoning (See p. 342)
- Ascertain which poison, and how much taken.
- Gastric aspiration and washout with saline if ingestion within six hours (not for paraffin, petrol, strong acids or alkalis).
- Do not induce vomiting.
- Give milk as universal antidote.
- Give activated charcoal 5–10 g in 100 ml water after gastric emptying.
- Educate parents to keep all poisons out of reach.

REFER
- All cases for observation and medical opinion.

Rheumatic fever (See p. 342)
- Bed rest.
- Aspirin (Disprin®): for fever and joint pains.

REFER
- All cases should be initially referred to hospital.

ACTION

- Penicillin V 250 mg, six-hourly for ten days.
- Weekly ESR to assess progress.
- Explain to parents importance of prophylactic monthly benzathine penicillin and regular follow-up.

- Before dental extraction or extensive fillings of teeth, child must go to hospital or see doctor, for special ampicillin prophylaxis.

Ringworm (See p. 300)
Body
- Apply Whitfield®'s ointment three times daily until cleared (may take several weeks).

Scalp
- As above, but add oral griseofulvin.
- Look for nits (may have accompanying pediculosis).

Scabies (See p. 301)
Benzyl Benzoate method (May burn)
- Wash body, cut nails.
- Dry well.
- Cover body with lotion (not face or head).
- Allow to dry and apply another layer.
- Dress.
- No washing for 24 hours.

REFER

- Not responding to therapy.

- Failure to respond.
- All cases where nails are affected.

ACTION	REFER

ACTION

- Then wash and put on new clothes and bedclothes.
- Or: gamma benzene hexachloride 1% (Lindane® / Quellada®) may be applied and left on for eight hours in children (not infants).

Or: Tetmosol® soap method
- Wash body, cover in lather.
- Leave on to dry.
- Dress.
- Repeat procedure next day.
- Leave soap on for another 24 hours.
- Wash all clothes and bedding with soap.

Or: 2,5% sulphur ointment
- Children under 6 months: Apply three times a day for three days.

Shock (Hypovolaemic) (See p. 163)
- Immediate IV Haemaccel®, Plasmalyte or normal saline 20 mg/kg rapidly.
- Sodium bicarbonate 8%, IV 2 ml/kg.
- Oxygen.
- Blood glucose (reagent strip).
- Monitor urine output (urine bag).
- If shock persists, repeat Haemaccel®/plasma, etc. 10 ml/kg.

REFER

- All cases.

ACTION

- Once BP established, continue IV therapy with half-Dextrose/Darrows solution.
- Stabilise before transferring.

Stridor (See p. 287)
- Co-trimoxazole or amoxicillin for five days.
- Anti-fever measures.
- Moisten air around child with steam if possible.
- If cyanosis, give oxygen.
- Always consider foreign body.
- See again; not later than following day.
- Inform parents what to watch out for.

Note: Most cases should be referred to hospital

Squint (See p. 254)
- Refer all cases to the nearest eye clinic or hospital and explain importance of this to parents.

Trauma
Lacerations (See p. 322)
- Clean and suture if necessary.
- Tetanus toxoid if indicated.
- Antibiotic cover.
- Paracetamol for pain.
- Keep surrounding area clean.
- Check in two days and again later for removal of sutures.

REFER

- If stridor is both inspiratory and expiratory.
- Recession.
- Alar flare.
- Cyanosis.
- Restless.
- Tachypnoea.
- Feeding difficulty.
- Severely ill.

- All cases.
- Sudden onset: Urgently.
- Long history: Non-urgent

- If underlying tissue damage suspected, e.g. to tendons; or in case of fractures or deep penetrating wound.

ACTION

- Child to be seen any time for rise in temperature or other signs of infection.

  Fractures *(See p. 320)*
- Paracetamol.

Whooping cough *(See p. 239)*
- Antibiotic erythromycin, ampicillin or amoxicillin.
- Cough suppressant, e.g. Nitepax®.
- Oxygen if needed.
- Full blood count if diagnosis uncertain.
- Another feed after vomiting (usually retained).
- See again at intervals.

REFER

- Refer all cases for further assessment and X-ray.

- Respiratory distress.
- Apnoeic spells.
- Cyanotic spells.
- Convulsions.
- Dehydration / severe vomiting.

Commonly used medications and dosage guidelines

Antibiotics
- Amoxicillin dosage using a 125 mg /5 ml suspension:

Table C.1

Age	Weight	Amoxicillin 125 mg per 5 ml given three times a day
2–12 months	3 to under 6 kg	5 ml
	6 to under 10 kg	7,5 ml
12–60 months	10–25 kg	12,5 ml

- Co-trimoxazole (Bactrim®, Septran®, Purbac®);
  ○ Over six weeks and under six months: 2,5 ml twice daily.
  ○ Six months to five years: 5 ml twice daily.
  ○ Six to 12 years: 10 ml twice daily.
  ○ Over 12 years: Two tablets twice daily.
- Co-trimoxazole prophylaxis for PJP (PCP) pneumonia – use in HIV-exposed children over six weeks of age for the first year of life and for older children with symptomatic HIV infection.

Table C.2

Weight	Dose of co-trimoxazole suspension given three times a week
Under 5 kg	5 ml
5–10 kg	7,5 ml
11–15 kg	10 ml
Over 15 kg	15 ml

- Erythromycin (Ilosone®, Erythrocin®, etc.);
  ○ 25–50 mg/kg/day: Given in four divided doses.

Table C.3 Dosage using a 125 mg/5 ml suspension

Age	Weight	Erythromycin 125 mg/5 ml given four times a day
2–36 months	8 to under 10 kg	2,5ml
	10 to under18 kg	5ml
36–60 months	18 to under 25 kg	10ml

- Metronidazole (Flagyl®) (for giardiasis) syrup contains 200 mg/5 ml.
  ○ 7 mg/kg/dose given orally eight-hourly for seven days.

Table C.4 Metronidazole doses to be given eight-hourly

Weight	Approx age	Dose mg	Suspension 200 mg/5 ml one hour before food	Tablet 200 mg with or after food	Tablet 400 mg with or after food
3–6	0–3 months	40 mg	1 ml	-	-
6–10	3–12 months	80 mg	2 ml	-	-
10–18	1–5 years	120 mg	3 ml	-	-
18–25	5–8 years	200 mg	5 ml	1 tablet	½ tablet
25–50	8–14 years	400 mg	–	2 tablets	1 tablet

- Nalidixic acid (urinary tract infection):
  ○ Not recommended under three months of age.
  ○ Dose is 50 mg/kg/day: In divided doses given four times daily.

Using a 250 mg/5 ml suspension, the doses to be given four times a day are:
  ○ 2–5 years 250 mg/dose: 5 ml.
  ○ Over 5 years 375 mg/dose: 7,5ml.

- Penicillin V suspension:
  - Under 6 months: 125 mg four times daily.
  - 6 months to 10 years: 250 mg four times daily.
- Penicillin V tablets:
  - Over six years: 250 mg tablets four times daily.
  - Much less expensive than suspension.

Anti-TB drugs
See employing authority directions.

Anticonvulsants
- Phenobarbitone (elixir / tablets):
  - 5–10 mg/kg/day (maximum 120 mg/day): Single dose at night or by day.
- Phenytoin (Epanutin®) (suspension / tabs / caps):
  - 15 mg/kg dose twice daily.
- Diazepam (Valium®): See Emergency drugs.

Antifungal / Antimonilial
- Whitfield®'s ointment.
- 2% Miconazole cream.
- Nystatin (Mycostatin®) suspension 100 000 units/ml:
  - 0,5 ml in mouth, four times daily, after feed.
- Nystatin ointment for skin lesions / nappy area:
  - Also works well in oral monilia.

Antihelmintics *(For parasites)*
- Albendazole (Zentel® tabs) – broad spectrum:
  - Under two years: 200 mg single dose
  - Older than two years: 400 mg single dose
- Mebendazole (Vermox® tabs / suspension):
  - One tablet twice daily for three days (all ages) for round worms.
  - 5 ml twice daily for three days (infants).
  - **Note**: For tapeworms: 12-hourly for six days 100 mg .

Antihistamines
- Hydroxyzine (Aterax®):
  - Infants 0,5 mg/kg/dose (drops) divided doses 12-hourly orally.
  - Children 0,5-1 mg/kg/dose (syrup) 12-hourly orally.
  - Use with caution in children under six years.

- Promethazine elixir (Phenergan®) 5 mg/5 ml:
  - Dose: 0,1 mg/kg/dose eight-hourly.

Antipyretics
- Paracetamol (Panado®):
  - Given four times daily.
  - Under one year: 2,5 ml/dose.
  - One to three years: 2,5–5 ml/dose.
  - Three to six years: 5 ml/dose.
  - Six to 12 years: Half tablet/dose.

Bronchodilators
- Salbutamol (Ventolin®):
  - 0,15 mg/kg/dose: Given four times daily.
  - Metered Dose Inhaler (MDI) with spacer one to two puffs six-hourly.
  - Nebuliser liquid: Use 1 ml mixed with 1 ml normal saline for each treatment.

Cough preparations
- Cough Linctus:
  - Under six months: 2,5 ml eight-hourly.
  - Over six months: 5 ml eight-hourly.

Decongestants
- Decongestant mixture (e.g. Actifed® / Demazin® / Dimetapp®):
  - Under 1 year: 1,25–2,5 ml six-hourly.
  - One to three years: 2,5–5 ml six-hourly.
  - Over three years: 5 ml six-hourly.
- Iliadin® nose drops:
  - **Note:** Do not use for longer than three days.
- NaBic nose drops.
- Normal saline nose drops.

Eardrops
- Boric acid drops.
- Acetic acid drops.

Emergency drugs
- Adrenaline (bronchospasm / anaphylaxis):
  - 0,01 ml/kg/dose: Maximum 0,5 ml subcutaneous.
- Valium® (convulsions):
  Intravenous dose:
  - 0,3 mg/kg (maximum 10 mg) IV: Slowly over two minutes.
  Rectal Doses:
  - 0,5 mg/kg (maximum 10 mg).
  - If convulsion not terminated after the initial dose, half the dose can be repeated after ten minutes. Not recommended under one month; use phenobarbitone.

Table C.5 Rectal dosage of diazepam

Weight	Age	Using Valium® (diazepam) 10 mg in 2 ml
3 to under 4 kg	2–6 months	2 mg (0,4 ml)
4 to under 5 kg	2–6 months	2,5 mg (0,5 ml)
5 to under 15 kg	6–24 months	5 mg (1 ml)
15 to under 25 kg	24–60 months	7,5 mg (1,5 ml)

- Activated charcoal (poisoning / drug over dosage):
  - 1 g/kg in 100 ml water.

Eye ointments / drops
- Chloramphenicol ointment.
- Tetracycline ointment.

Skin preparations
- Aqueous cream.
- Ascabiol® (Benzyl benzoate).
- Betadine cream / ointment / shampoo.
- Calamine lotion.
- GBH Lotion (gamma benzene hexachloride 1%).
- 1% hydrocortisone / HEB (HEB is an emulsifying ointment).
- 1% hydrocortisone / zinc / nystatin.
- 10% steroid/HEB (short-term use only).

- 5% sulphur.
- Mercurochrome.
- Mycostatin® cream/ointment.
- Tetmosol® soap.
- Whitfield®'s ointment.
- Zinc and castor oil.
- Zinc and Vioform.

Tonics / Vitamins

- Multivitamin drops: 0,6 ml daily.
- Multivitamin syrup: 5 ml daily.
- Ferrodrops®: 0,3–0,6 ml daily.
- Ferrous sulphate (BPC): 300 mg per 5 ml (60 mg elemental iron in 5 ml):
  - Therapeutic: 6 mg (elemental iron)/kg/day.
  - Prophylactic: 1 mg (elemental iron)/kg/day.
  - Both in three divided doses/day.

Other

- Prednisone (usually 1 mg/kg/day or less).

Dose to be given once daily for seven to ten days for persistent asthmatic wheeze.

For stridor, a single dose is given prior to urgent referral to hospital.

Table C.6 Prednisone dosages

Weight	Prednisone 5mg tablets
4–6 kg	2 tablets
6–9 kg	3 tablets
9–12 kg	4 tablets
12–14 kg	5 tablets
14–17 kg	6 tablets
17–19 kg	7 tablets
19–20 kg	8 tablets

- Sorol / other ORS (Oral Rehydration Solution) sachets.
- Lignocaine in tannic acid jelly (oral herpes).
- Colic mixture.

Please note: Page numbers in italics refer to
tables and figures.